Risking Antimicrobial Resistance

Carsten Strøby Jensen
Søren Beck Nielsen • Lars Fynbo
Editors

Risking Antimicrobial Resistance

A collection of one-health studies of antibiotics and its social and health consequences

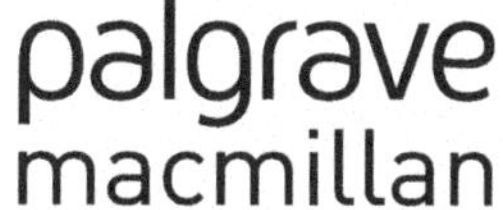

Editors
Carsten Strøby Jensen
Department of Sociology
University of Copenhagen
Copenhagen, Denmark

Lars Fynbo
VIVE – The Danish Center for Social Science Research
Copenhagen, Denmark

Søren Beck Nielsen
Department of Nordic Studies and Linguistics
University of Copenhagen
Copenhagen, Denmark

ISBN 978-3-030-08067-9 ISBN 978-3-319-90656-0 (eBook)
https://doi.org/10.1007/978-3-319-90656-0

Softcover re-print of the Hardcover 1st edition 2019

Cover illustration: © Caiaimage/Andy Roberts
Cover design: Tom Howey

Printed on acid-free paper

This Palgrave Macmillan imprint is published by the registered company Springer International Publishing AG part of Springer Nature.
The registered company address is: Gewerbestrasse 11, 6330 Cham, Switzerland

Preface

Antimicrobial resistance (AMR) has become one of the twenty-first century's major health challenges. Since World War II, antimicrobials have been widely used to fight bacterial diseases in humans. Diseases that were once serious and sometimes fatal to humans could be cured or prevented using antimicrobials. However, the successful use of antimicrobials has also had a drawback. Each and every time antimicrobials are used, these create a risk that the bacteria being treated will develop resistance. Antimicrobials, therefore, have become less and less effective over time, and antimicrobial resistance (AMR) has emerged as one of our major health risks.

In *Risking Antimicrobial Resistance*, we have set out to analyze the development of AMR within an explicitly social science perspective. While AMR can be seen as belonging fundamentally to the health sciences area, its development, its risks, and the public debate surrounding AMR are replete with important social science issues. For example, there are major differences among countries in the amount of antibiotics used to treat the same types of diseases. These national differences in consumption have little to do with the actual epidemiology of infections and are more indicative of differences between countries in terms of habits, culture, legislation, and economics.

This book is the result of a research project at the University of Copenhagen, entitled 'UC-care' (University of Copenhagen Center for

Control of Antibiotic Resistance). The Center is a multidisciplinary research center that brings together researchers from many departments across the university. The UC-Care project was launched by the University of Copenhagen in 2012 as part of the university's enhanced focus on interdisciplinary cooperation on selected key issues. Hence, UC-Care involved researchers from the health sciences, veterinary science, social sciences, and the humanities. This book presents some of the results of the social and humanities part of the project, and the authors are all affiliated with UC-Care and the University of Copenhagen.

In connection with the book, there are a number of people we wish to thank. First, we wish to thank Professor Luca Guardabassi of the University of Copenhagen and Ross University's School of Veterinary Medicine. Having taken the initiative for the UC-Care project, Professor Guardabassi has been instrumental in obtaining funds for carrying out the research for this book. We also wish to thank Professor Anders Miki Bojesen of the University of Copenhagen for his work as Principal Investigator in the second half of the UC-Care project. We also express our gratitude to our fellow UC-Care participants from the health and veterinary fields for their enthusiastic cooperation with those of us from the social sciences and humanities.

We also wish to express our thanks to the many interviewees and participants (notably patients and doctors) who, as described in the chapters of the book, kindly agreed to be interviewed, observed, or video-recorded by the researchers involved. Overall, the book's chapters are based on interviews with more than 200 people. This research could not have been accomplished without the active participation of the Interviewees, and for this we are extremely grateful.

Our book has been improved by the anonymous reviewers who commented on each of the chapters in the book. Their efforts are highly appreciated.

In completing the manuscript, we wish to thank Anna Gørting Jensen and Steven Sampson. Anna Gørting Jensen helped in editing the manuscript and keeping track of the individual chapters. Steven Sampson's language editing helped in ensuring that our ideas could be expressed in the best possible English.

Finally, we wish to thank Palgrave for being willing to publish the book and for their patience during the process of completing the manuscript.

Any defects in the book, of course, are solely our own.

Copenhagen, Denmark — Carsten Strøby Jensen
Copenhagen, Denmark — Søren Beck Nielsen
Copenhagen, Denmark — Lars Fynbo
January 2018

Contents

Notes on Contributors

Mads Bank holds a Ph.D. in Psychology from the University of Copenhagen and is currently teaching personality psychology and educational psychology at the University of Copenhagen, The University of Aarhus and The University of Southern Denmark. His research focuses on how professionals learn, work, and organize their practices in organisations working with health, social work, and education. More specifically, his research draws on governmentality studies in order to analyse how professionals in a welfare society develop and educate citizens and co-workers. Recent publications include "Beyond spaces of counselling, Qualitative Social Work" (With Nissen, M.), in Qualitative Social Work, 2017; and "Enacting (Post) Psychological Standards in Social Work: From regimes of visibility to user-driven standards & affective subjectification, Theory & Psychology" in Theory & Psychology, 2016.

Lars Fynbo is researcher at VIVE – The Danish Center for Social Science Research, Denmark. He holds a Ph.D. in Sociology. He works in a cross-over between Welfare Studies and Cultural Sociology. His research primarily focuses on risk behavior in a symbolic interactionist perspective. Lars also lectures at the Department of Public Health and the Department of Sociology, University of Copenhagen. His recent publications include "Analysing the significance of silence in qualitative interviewing: questioning and shifting power relations" in Qualitative Research, 2017 and "Immoral, deviant, or just normal: Drunk drivers' narratives of drinking and drunk driving" in Contemporary Drug Problems, 2014.

Nieves Hernández-Flores is Associate Professor at the Department of English, Germanics and Romance Studies, University of Copenhagen. Her primary area of research includes relations between language and society in the Spanish speaking countries and her research mainly concentrates on pragmatics, politeness and *face* studies, discourse and identity, discourse and ideology, interculturalism, and media studies. Recent publications include "Lo que se debe hacer es cambiar un poco el estilo de vida. Estrategias de atenuación en el consejo médico" (with Rodríguez-Tembrás, Vanesa) in *Spanish in Context*, 2018; "El papel del acopañante en la consulta médica atención primaria. Roles y efectos sociales" in *Oralia*, 201; and "Barbara De Cock (2014). Profiling Discourse Participants. Forms and functions in Spanish conversation and debates" in *revue Romane*, 2016.

Carsten Strøby Jensen is Associate Professor at the Department of Sociology, University of Copenhagen. He holds an M.A. in Cultural Sociology and a Ph.D. (dr.scient.soc.) in Sociology, from the University of Copenhagen. He has been head of research on the 'Risking Antimicrobial Resistance' project. His research mainly focuses on political sociology, employment relations, and medical sociology. He has a specific interest in the theoretical development of theories relating to European integration, for example, in connection with the development of health policy in EU. During the last four years, he has worked more intensively within the field of medical sociology, especially with a focus on antimicrobial consumption and antimicrobial resistance. He has been involved in research management for many years and has been a member of the research management committee in the UC-care project. He has published in journals like 'Social Science & Medicine'.

Kim Sune Jepsen is a doctoral student at the Department of Sociology, Lund University. He holds a B.A. and M.A. in Sociology from the University of Copenhagen and an M.A. in Society Technology Nature from Lancaster University. His research interests include the changing value of labour in post-socialist capitalism in Central and Eastern Europe. The primary aim of his research is to identify the subjective experiences and critical trajectories of working life within a radical change from socialism to flexible forms of capitalism, thus, exploring the thesis that 'new spirits of capitalism' are emerging in CEE. His recent publications include "Cochlear Implantation : Exploring Technoscience and Designs on Citizenship" in *The International Library of Ethics, Law and Technology*, Springer, 2017; "Wired to freedom: Life Science, public politics and the case of Cochlear Implantation" in *Public Understanding of Science*, 2017; and "'The public Spectre': A critical Concept of Public Engagement with Technology" (with Delgado, Ana; Bertilsson, Margareta) in *Technoscience and Citizenship: Ethics and Governance in the Digital Society*, Springer, 2017.

Kirsten A. Jeppesen Kragh is Head of Studies at the Department of English, Germanics and Romance studies, University of Copenhagen. She holds a Ph.D. in French Linguistics and is Associate Professor of French language at the Department of English, Germanics and Romance studies, University of Copenhagen. Her fields of interests are research and education policy, particularly focusing on foreign language and strengthening of the foreign language studies and their roots in the interaction between language and culture. Her research domains are language change, functional grammar, linguistic variation, and paradigmatic and constructional change, and her current research concentrates on perception verbs and their complementation, infinitive syntax, deictic relative clauses, modal variation after perception verbs and verbs of utterance, and temporal marking of subjunctive forms. Recent publications include "Hvad kan en funktionel og variationistisk grammatik tilføre beskrivelsen af det franske sprog?" (with Kragh, Kirsten A. Jeppesen; Lindschouw, Jan Juhl; Hansen, Anita Berit) in Ny forskning I grammatik 24, 2017; "Derfor har vi brug for paradigmer" (with Kragh, Kirsten A. Jeppesen; Schøsler, Lene) in Forskning i ny Grammatik, 2016, and "Les variations diasystématiques et leurs interdépendances dans les langues romanes" (with Lindschouw, Jan Juhl).

Johanna Lindell is lecturer at the Department of Nordic Studies and Linguistics, University of Copenhagen. Johanne holds an M.A. in Psychology of Language from the University of Copenhagen and a Ph.D. in Health Communication. Her research concentrates on Conversation Analysis and doctor–patient communication. Her recent research projects include *Reducing Resistance: Communication and treatment decisions on antibiotics in Danish primary care*, University of Copenhagen, The Department of humanities, 2017; "Overvej en ekstra gang hvad du siger til lægen!" (with Nielsen, Søren Beck) in *Forskerzonen*, 2017; "Antibiotika I almen praksis. En fælles beslutning?" in *Akademisk Kvarter*, 2015; and "Interaktionens betydning for nedsættelse af antibiotikaforbrug: Et konversationsanalytisk singe-case studie af design af behandlingsforslag i almen praksis" in *NyS*, 2015.

Søren Beck Nielsen is Associate Professor at the Department of Nordic Studies and Linguistics, University of Copenhagen where he teaches the subject psychology of language and is a member of the research centre Intersubjectivity in Medical Communication (Inmedic). His main research area is oral health communication. Using conversation analysis, he has investigated various types of communication in health care encounters, notably in geriatric wards and in general practice. These studies have elucidated the conversational procedures by which participants, for example, produce and use medical records; open up and close down consultations; make important decisions accountable, and so on. Recent publications include: 'If you don't get better, you may come back here': proposing conditioned follow-ups to the doctor's office in Text & Talk 2018, How doctors manage consulting computer records while interacting with patients in Research on Language and Social Interaction 2016; Medical record keeping as interactional accomplishment in Pragmatics and Society 2014.

Sandi Michele de Oliveira is Associate Professor at the Department of English, Germanic and Romance studies. She holds an M.A. in Foreign Language Education—Portuguese and English and a Ph.D. in Foreign Language Education—Specialization in Applied Linguistics; both from the University of Texas. She has a history as Assistant Professor at the Department of Linguistics and Literature, University of Évora, Portugal. The unifying theme encompassing most of her research is the way speakers construct identities through discourse, a topic that brings together sociolinguistics, pragmatics, discourse analysis, communities of practice, and interaction analysis. Projects within this broad theme include address forms, politeness, political discourse, and strategic communication for those living in border communities or transnational situations. Her recent publications include: "Discourse of Inclusion and Exclusion in the Commemoration of the 40th Anniversary of the Portuguese Revolution" in *Journal of Social Science Education*, 2015; and "Interpretative challenges in face analysis" (with Hernández-Flores, Nieves) in *Textos en Proceso*, 2015.

Inge Kryger Pedersen is Associate Professor at the Department of Sociology, University of Copenhagen. She holds an M.A. in Cultural Sociology and a Ph.D. in Sociology from the University of Copenhagen. Her research concentrates on health-related issues concerning forms of knowledge and practice within medical technologies. Her analyses concern how actors and professionals seek to optimize different forms of bodily practice and expertise. She applies perspectives of sociology of knowledge and culture in examining knowledge-creating institutions such as medicine and health technology. She is the co-director of the departmental research group *Knowledge, Organization and Politics* and a co-promotor to the recent opening of the *Centre for the Sociological Study of Science, Expertise and Society* (CEVES). Her teaching areas are general sociology, social theory, sociology of health, methodology, and methods. Relevant publications include "The emergence of trust in clinics of alternative medicine" (with Hansen, V.H.; Grüneberg, k. Jan), in *Sociology of Health and Illness*, 2016; "'It can do no harm': Body maintenance and modification in alternative medicine acknowledged as a non-risk health regimen" in *Social Science & Medicine*, 2013; "'Fantastic hands'—but no evidence: The construction of expertise by users of CAM" (with C. Baarts), in *Social Science & Medicine*, 2010; and "Doping and the perfect body expert: social and cultural indicators of performance-enhancing drug use in Danish gyms" in *Sport in Society*, 2010.

Vanesa Rodríguez-Tembrás lectures at the Institute for Translation and Interpretation and the Department of Romance Languages, University of Heidelberg. She holds an M.A. in Literature from Complutense University of Madrid. Her research concentrates on pragmatics, sociolinguistics, and language identity in Spanish and Galician. Currently, she is writing her dissertation about mitigation as a pragmatic strategy in doctor–patient communication in Galician and Spanish. Her recent publications include "Lo que se debe hacer es cambiar un poco el estilo de vida. Estrategias de atenuación en el consejo médico" (with Hernández Flores, Nieves) in Spanish in Context, 2018 and "Alternancia de lenguas como estrategia de actividad de imagen en la comunicación médico-paciente en un consultorio gallego" in TEP. Textos en Proceso, 2016.

Anne Rogne is working as counselor and coordinator at 'Psykologisk korttidsrådgivning' Copenhagen. She works at the Nordic organization, Falck, as psychological telephone counselor and as student assistant at REforM, Aarhus University. Anne holds a B.A. in Medicine and Psychology and an M.A. in Psychology; both from the University of Copenhagen. Anne has previously worked as Teaching Assistant, at the Department of Psychology, teaching social psychological theory and methods. She has also worked as editor of the Student Magazine *Indput*.

Erling Strudsholm is Associate Professor at the Department of English, Germanic and Romance Studies, University of Copenhagen. He holds an M.A. in Italian and a Ph.D. in Italian Language, from the University of Copenhagen. His research concentrates on sociolinguistics, language variation, contrastive linguistics, perception verbs, idiomatic expressions with numbers and colour words, deixis, and pronouns. His recent publications include "Color words in Danish and Italian idioms" (with Bazzanella, Carla; Ronga, Irene) in Color language and color categorization, Cambridge Scholars Press, 2016; "Åbninger og lukninger i emailkorrespondance på fire sprog" (with Skafte Jensen, Eva; Kragh, Kirsten A. Jeppesen) in Globe: A journal of language, culture and communication, 2016; "Metaphors and emotion in colour words" (with Bazzanella, Carla;

Ronga, Irene) in Colour and colour naming: Crosslinguistic approaches, Centro de Linguística da Universidade de Lisboa/Universidade de Aveiro, 2016; "Quattro gatti e una mosca bianca: Espressioni con nomi di animali in una prospettiva comparativa italiano-danese in Parole, gesti, interpretazioni: Studi linguistici per Carla Bazzanella. 2015; and "Verbi di percezione come segnali discorsivi" in Testualità: Fondamenti, unità, relazioni. Ferrari, A., Lala, L. & Stojomenova, R. (red.). Franco Cesati Editore, 2015.

List of Tables

1

Risking Antimicrobial Resistance: A One Health Study of Antibiotic Use and Its Societal Aspects

Carsten Strøby Jensen, Søren Beck Nielsen, and Lars Fynbo

1.1 Introduction

Antimicrobial resistance is one of the twenty-first century's greatest health challenges. In a number of reports, the World Health Organization (WHO) has emphasized how the development of antibiotic resistance will be on the increase as a consequence of the excessive consumption of antibiotics within healthcare and in livestock farming. In a number of

C. S. Jensen (✉)
Department of Sociology, University of Copenhagen, Copenhagen, Denmark
e-mail: csj@soc.ku.dk

S. B. Nielsen
Department of Nordic Studies and Linguistics, University of Copenhagen, Copenhagen, Denmark
e-mail: sbnielsen@hum.ku.dk

L. Fynbo
VIVE – The Danish Center for Social Science Research, Copenhagen, Denmark
e-mail: lafy@vive.dk

C. S. Jensen et al. (eds.), *Risking Antimicrobial Resistance*,
https://doi.org/10.1007/978-3-319-90656-0_1

articles, *The Lancet* has discussed issues related to antibiotics and presented similar warnings. In November 2013, *The Lancet* wrote:

> The causes of antibiotic resistance are complex and include human behaviour at many levels of society; the consequences affect everybody in the world. … Antibiotics paved the way for unprecedented medical and societal developments, and are today indispensible in all health systems … Within just a few years, we might be faced with dire setbacks, medically, socially, and economically, unless real and unprecedented global coordinated actions are immediately taken.

Based on contemporary research from the social sciences and humanities, this anthology elucidates the antibiotic resistance issue from a range of scientific perspectives. Such a cross-disciplinary contribution has been missing in the debates about use of antibiotics and the development of antibiotic-resistant pathogenic bacteria. The contributors to this book include sociologists, political scientists, psychologists, and linguists, reflecting expertise within a wide range of social sciences and humanities.

There are three main, recurring perspectives in the anthology: (1) 'One Health', (2) the Danish context, and (3) the social and human perspectives.

1.1.1 One Health

The One Health perspective has won ground within both the veterinary and human medical sciences during the last ten to 15 years. As a consequence, the former professional division into veterinary and human medical paradigms has now been increasingly replaced by a shared paradigm now known as 'One Health'. The One Health perspective reflects advances in our understanding of how human and veterinary biological processes resemble and interact with each other. For example, a large proportion of the recently discovered pathogens (both harmful bacteria and harmful vira) derive from the transfer of vira or bacteria between people and animals. These zoonoses (i.e. infectious diseases of animals that can be transmitted to humans) have put the One Health perspective on the agenda of veterinary and human medical research. With regard to the development of resistance to antibiotics, this problem is known from the special type of resistant bacteria designated as Methicillin-Resistant *Staphylococcus aureus* (MRSA). MRSA is a strain of *Staphylococcus aureus* that has developed resistance to the most common type of antibiotic used, that is, methicillin (Methicillin-Resistant *Staphylococcus aureus*). A specific variation of these resistant bacteria, called MRSA-398, spreads from pigs to humans, and it is MRSA-398 resistance that has drawn considerable international attention. The One Health perspective thus plays a central role in this book: some chapters focus on the human area, others on the veterinary, and some of the chapters combine the two, examining, for example, the governance mechanisms that seek to regulate the two areas. The development (and prevention) of antimicrobial resistance is thus seen as a problem related to both the human and veterinary areas, and it must therefore be viewed in this One Health context.

1.1.2 The Danish Context

The second key perspective of the analysis is geographical. Our book focuses mainly on Denmark and on the development of resistance in Denmark. Our book originates from a Danish research project, and takes this as its natural starting point. The background to the focus on Denmark, however, is not just expedient. Denmark, like the other Nordic countries, is characterized by a significantly lower general level of antibiotic resistance than many other countries. This low level of resistance distinguishes Denmark from both other European countries and from the rest of the world. Moreover, Denmark is also a country with significant veterinary production. For example, around 30 million pigs are produced annually, and pig farming accounts for a large proportion of Denmark's antibiotics consumption. Part of the reason for Denmark's relatively low level of resistance derives from Danish authorities' high level of attention paid to the development of resistance in the human sector. Hence, Danish authorities have sought to limit the use of antibiotics—especially during the last ten years—by, for instance, preparing guidelines for physicians and patients so as to ensure rational and responsible use of antibiotics. A number of initiatives in the veterinary area have also been launched in order to limit use of antibiotics in this sector as well. These initiatives include schemes to monitor the veterinary sector's use of antibiotics right down to the individual farm level, distributed by type of livestock, type of antibiotic, and so on. This kind of monitoring has been one way in which Denmark has been able to control the development of resistance. Several of the book's chapters describe how antibiotics are used (or avoided) in a Danish context. Questions raised are, for example, 'Under what circumstances do Danish doctors prescribe antibiotics to their patients?' 'Do Danish prescription practices differ from those in Southern Europe?' 'Are Danish doctors more or less prone than doctors in other countries to "give in" to patients' requests to receive antibiotic treatment?' These are just some of the questions that the articles in this anthology address. Other chapters are case studies describing how the risk posed by antibiotics is interpreted by various social groups in Danish society. In Denmark, and also internationally, considerable disagreement can be observed between, for example, representatives of the veterinary sector and the human sector regarding primary responsibility for the increase in antibiotic resistance. In the veterinary sector, it is often argued that it is primarily the human consumption of antibiotics that leads to resistance, while those working in the human sector point to the effects of antibiotics consumption in pig farming as the key factor behind the development of resistance. In order to underscore the comparative perspective in this book, a number of chapters focus on analysing the use of antibiotics in France, Italy and Spain. Here, focus is especially on the relations between patients and physicians in the primary health care sector. These chapters utilize case studies of interactions between patients and physicians in the three countries.

1.1.3 The Social and Human Perspectives

The book's third overall perspective is related to how the analyses are based primarily on social science and humanities research traditions. The authors of the individual chapters are all researchers with backgrounds in the social sciences and/or the humanities. In this respect, the book differs from most other publications concerning antibiotic resistance, which are traditionally dominated by researchers with medical or veterinary orientations. The reason for this social scientific and humanities focus is that an understanding of antibiotic resistance can by no means be described in terms of purely biological or biomedical processes. The development of resistance is highly dependent on the way in which antibiotics are used in a given society. And the users are, of course, humans, who either request them from doctors, dispense them to patients, or feed them to their farm animals. The fact that, as indicated above, the development of resistance in Denmark (and in the Nordic region) is at a lower level than other European Union (EU) countries in the EU is primarily related to the societal context in which antibiotics are used. It should be noted that the 'medical' instructions (whether this is in the veterinary or human sector) for administration of antibiotics are the same for Denmark as for other countries. The difference lies in the societal context in which the use of antibiotics takes place. It is these social processes which affect the way antibiotics are dispensed and consumed and thereby the probability of resistance being developed. The chapters and cases described in this book focus especially on two aspects of antibiotics consumption. One aspect concerns what is called the relation between 'prescribers' and 'users' of antibiotics. In the international literature, we have descriptions of how the relation between prescribers (e.g. physicians and veterinary surgeons) and users (e.g. patients or farmers) in itself affects the way antibiotics are used. Physicians may feel pressure to prescribe antibiotics for sick children if their parents are worried, even though the child probably has a viral infection against which antibiotics will have little effect (Stivers 2007). The veterinary surgeon may experience how farmers solicit preventive treatment for their pig herd, even though the herd appears to be completely healthy. The interaction between 'prescribers' and 'users' is analysed in a number of the book's chapters. The other key social science aspect concerns what can be termed the regulatory or governmental perspective. The use of antibiotics is embedded in a governmental and regulatory context that has a direct effect on society's overall use of antibiotics. Within the EU, for example, antibiotics may generally only be sold on prescription, irrespective of whether they are used in the human or veterinary sector. Globally, on the other hand, this is by no means always the case. In a number of countries (such as India and Pakistan), antibiotics are sold over the counter. There may be numerous reasons for regulatory differences from one country to another, but the consequences are clear. In some parts of Pakistan and India, the consumption of antibiotics is very significant, and the development of resistance is high. The regulatory regime thus affects the use of antibiotics and the tendency for high levels of resistance to develop. In this light, this book focuses especially on the governmental structures that dominate in Denmark, as well as on the extent to which these structures affect antibiotics consumption in both the veterinary and human sectors. The aim is to contribute to an international understanding of the relationship between regulation, antibiotics consumption, and the development of resistance. In this context, Denmark represents a highly relevant case, since it has managed to maintain a low level of antimicrobial resistance (AMR) compared to other countries while still ensuring a high standard of healthcare. In addition, pig farming is a major sector of the Danish agricultural economy and is internationally competitive. Even though there is some national scepticism towards the risk of the development of resistance due to the intensive pig production, the pig-raising sector's consumption of antibiotics is lower than comparable production units in other countries. In some of the book's chapters, therefore, focus is on explaining the nature of the mechanisms that make it possible to maintain highly effective and extensive pig production while also seeking to limit the use of antibiotics.

1.2 The Concept of Risk

Another central perspective in the book relates to the concept of risk and to the question of what in late modern society is perceived as risky behaviour. Within the social sciences, the concept of risk has been prominent for quite a few years, and a number of researchers have described how late modern society can be characterized as a risk society. The risk perspective is also relevant to the issue of antimicrobials and the development of AMR. In this context, the risk perspective can contribute to the analysis in at least two ways. First, it can elucidate the discussion of what can be termed the actual risk, posing the question: What actual risks does the development of AMR pose for the health and disease of people (and animals)? A post-antibiotic society will be affected by diseases that had been viewed as relatively harmless since the mid-1950s, diseases which, because of AMR, again become serious and in many situations life-threatening (Bonilla and Muniz 2009; Drlica and Perlin 2011; Podolsky 2006, 2015). A second benefit of the risk perspective concerns the issue of how antibiotics and the development of resistance are interpreted in society in general and among society's stakeholders in particular. Risk assessments are always embedded in an interpretative context that can be viewed as a social construction. This is apparent when physicians in the human sector often blame the veterinary sector for the development of resistance among humans, while stakeholders in the veterinary sector respond that the development of resistance has evolved primarily due to the use of antimicrobials in the human sector.

Risk assessments are often part of a social context that affects how a given risk is described and conceptualized. Overall, risk is conceived as either 'realistic' (climate change causes floods, use of antimicrobials causes AMR, etc.) or as a 'social construction' (Bengtsson et al. 2015). For instance, studying the relationship between the use of antibiotics and the enhancement of resistant pathogens reflects the 'realist' conception of risk, while studying forms of governmentality is more reflective of the constructionist conception of risk.

In this context, we will focus especially on two theoretical perspectives within risk analysis and apply them to the analysis of antimicrobials and AMR. The first perspective takes its point of departure on Ulrich Beck's concept of risk society. The second perspective takes its point of departure in Michel Foucault's work on governmentality. Both perspectives contribute to our understanding of how antimicrobial consumption and AMR is perceived in the global community.

1.2.1 AMR and the Risk Society

Ulrich Beck has worked with the concept of risk within a realist framework. In his *Risk Society*, Beck argues that risks are increasingly embedded in modern and late modern societies (Beck 1992, 2009). Furthermore, he argues that risks have increasingly become a consequence of the way the production of wealth (in a broad sense) takes place in late modern society. He writes, 'In advanced modernity, the social production of wealth is systematically accompanied by the social production of risks' (Beck 2009, p. 19).

For Beck, risks are produced as an outcome of the production of wealth. Pollution and climate change problems are among classical types of risks that develop due to the production of wealth and can be seen as a consequence of societal developments.

Beck distinguishes between what he calls 'danger' and 'risk' (Bengtsson et al. 2015, p. 9). In the pre-modern society, hazards and danger were also part of life. However, these dangers are not the kind of dangers we have today, which are a consequence of human behaviour. 'The risks and hazards of today differ in an essential way from the superficially similar ones in the Middle Ages through the global nature of their threat (people, animals, and plants) and through their modern causes. They are risks of modernization' (Beck 1992, p. 21).

According to Beck, risks in late modern society have three specific characteristics. Firstly, the risks of today tend to be global in their character. They cross borders and are embedded in a global community. Secondly, risks are characterized by their abstract character. The risks of today 'escape perception', as Beck writes. The third point made by Beck relates to how the conceptualisation of risks is embedded in expert communities and scientific systems. Due to the abstract nature of risks, it is experts and scientific communities who are charged with interpreting the scope and the nature of risks.

The first point made by Beck relates to the global character of risks. The risks of today are not embedded in specific countries or in specific social strata. The risks of today cross borders and traverse social distinctions. The effects of climate change are a result of human actions and are global in character. These effects cannot be isolated or restricted to specific countries. The potential threats from nuclear weapons related to the intensified conflicts between Western countries and Russia are also global in its character. No human will be left untouched if a nuclear war were to break out. In similar respects, pollution now crosses borders and social strata. As Beck once famously wrote, 'Poverty is hierarchic, smog is democratic' (Beck 1992, p. 36).

The second point stressed by Beck is that the forms of risks today are characterized by the fact that they 'escape perception'. Risks are not 'perceptible to the senses ... the risks of the civilization of today typically escape perception and are localized in the sphere of physical and chemical formulas (e.g. toxins in foodstuffs or the nuclear threat)' (Beck 1992, p. 21). Because the risks of today escape perception, we have no way of observing, perceiving or understanding them. If you encounter a crocodile while walking along the banks of the Nile, you immediately know that you are in danger. You can perceive the danger coming from the crocodile. If you are living in Western Europe, however, and you are exposed to radioactivity from an explosion in a nuclear plant in the Ukraine, you have no possibility of perceiving the danger. These kinds of risks 'escape perception'. Hence, modern types of risks such as climate change and pollution, while they threaten mankind, are not perceivable; the risks have an abstract character.

The fact that the risks in late modern societies escape our perception entails that experts and expert communities play a crucial role as discoverers or interpreters of risks. This is the third point made by Beck. Due to the abstract character of risks, the perception of risks in late modern society is mediated and interpreted by expert communities. It was only the experts in nuclear physics and meteorology who could identify the risks coming from the radioactive clouds that hit Europe when the Chernobyl nuclear plant exploded. Non-experts had no chance of identifying the risks of radioactivity. Expert communities are thus accorded a special role in the management of risks in late modern societies. Expert communities, however, view the world and its risks in their specific ways. And even expert communities have scientific controversies and scientific uncertainties (Arnoldi 2009, p. 85).

If we consider the area of antimicrobial consumption and AMR through the lens of Beck's 'risk society', a number of the points made by Beck are very useful. The overall development of consumption of antimicrobials and the development of AMR are closely connected to the production of wealth in late modern society in several ways. First, antimicrobials are themselves part of a value-producing system.

Antimicrobials are a commodity produced by companies that can increase their profits as sales go up. Production of antimicrobials contributes to the gross domestic products (GDPs) in the countries where it is produced. Secondly, antimicrobials are used to increase the welfare of citizens by reducing the consequences of bacterial infections. Antimicrobials can be used to effectively treat various infections and are thus life-prolonging. Antimicrobials make it possible to perform 'modern medicine' (e.g. hip and heart replacement) when used in a prophylactic manner. Thirdly, antimicrobials are used in modern food production in order to increase livestock productivity. Cows, swine, chickens, and so on receive antimicrobials to reduce infections and/or increase growth. The use of antimicrobials is an integral part of modern livestock production and a precondition for modern livestock and poultry production.

Beck's observation that 'the risks of today' have a global character is certainly relevant when we consider antimicrobial consumption and the spread of AMR. AMR is found in a variety of regions and countries in the world. The close correlation between the overall consumption of antimicrobials and AMR usually entails that countries with a high level of consumption also have a high level of AMR (European Commission 2015). However, AMR tends to be global in nature. AMR bacteria spread to the global community through food, by travellers, and through many other channels. Whenever a person, animal, or food product is moved from one area to another or from one part of the globe to another, there is a risk that AMR bacteria spread with it. AMR that develops in one region of the world will sooner or later move to other regions. And AMR also crosses social strata in the same way as Beck observed about smog. AMR, like smog, is thus 'democratic', in the sense that it spreads independently of people's social position.

AMR risk, with its global character, cannot be managed within the nation–state framework. Political initiatives implemented solely at the national level might reduce the development of AMR for a period, but AMR will eventually creep over the national borders. As a consequence of AMRs' transnational nature, a number of global political initiatives have been taken. The United Nations (UN) and WHO are among the global political institutions that have initiated 'action plans' to combat AMR. Similarly, AMR has been a topic at the Group of Seven (G7) meetings, and the EU has formulated action plans in order to reduce overall consumption of antimicrobials (European Commission 2011; World Health Organization 2014a, 2015). The strength of the global institutions is questionable, however, and it is doubtful whether the various actions plans can actually reduce the risks related to AMR.

Beck's insistence that today's risks 'escape perception' certainly applies to AMR. AMR and its associated risks are non-observable; they cannot be sensed or identified without the use of advanced methods of microbiology. AMR is first observable to humans when we contract a bacterial infection that cannot be treated with antimicrobials. A tourist who visits Pakistan or India (two countries with a high prevalence of AMR) will be unaware that he or she may bring home resistant bacteria. The neighbour living close to a pig farm will not know if he or she has been infected with MRSA-398 (a specific type of AMR) coming from pigs. In a similar way, a hospitalized patient in an Italian hospital will not be aware that he or she might become AMR just by staying at that hospital. Like other types of modern risks, AMR escapes perception. It is only through information coming from expert communities that ordinary citizens can learn about the risks coming from AMR.

In this respect, the scientific community plays an important role in communicating the risks of AMR to the public. Only AMR experts can assess the risks related to antimicrobial consumption. Even doctors or veterinarians, despite being experts in their own fields, are dependent on the risk assessments of microbiologists or epidemiologists to determine the extent of AMR risk. Science, however, is not unambiguous. Science has its own controversies and is often delayed or contentious in identifying or interpreting data. Arnoldi writes:

> The role of science when it comes to risks seems both problematic and paradoxical ... First, without science, no one would have any knowledge of a broad range of risks, and the technologies causing risks would not have come into existence. Second, public concerns about risks are often accompanied by a distrust of scientific assurances that the technologies are safe, and yet public concerns are in many cases based on the scientific finding. Third, science seems to produce as much uncertainty as certainty ... science generates as many vague indicators of unknown possibilities (risks) as it generates positive certainties. (Arnoldi 2009, p. 87)

Arnoldi's observations apply well to the scientific discussion of antimicrobials and AMR. Here we can observe related paradoxes. Without science, there would have been no antimicrobials to help fight bacterial infections. On the other hand, had there not been antimicrobials, AMR would not have evolved. Similarly, distrust of the scientific community can also be observed in relation to AMR. For example, epidemiologists insist that there is only a very slight risk of being infected with AMR from eating meat purchased in a supermarket, even though antimicrobial-resistant bacteria can be found in 25% to 50% of the meat sold. Public distrust of the scientific community might lead consumers to avoid buying meat due to a perceived risk of being infected with AMR.

A major scientific controversy within the field of AMR relates to debates about whether and to what extent AMR spreads from animals to humans: to what extent is AMR in the human body caused by the use of antimicrobials in livestock production? Are high levels of AMR in a given population a consequence of high levels of antimicrobial consumption in the human or/and in the veterinarian sector? Scientists seem to be unsure how to answer these questions, and the uncertainty is transformed into specific discourses that argue for or against the effects of the use of antimicrobials in livestock production. This is not only a discussion within science, of course. The debate rages between various coalitions of interests grouped largely around either the veterinarian sector or the human sector. Both groups use science (and scientific uncertainty) to legitimate their points of view.

One reason that MRSA has become such a huge theme both in the public and scientific discussions relates to the fact that it is an example of a clearer causal link between the use of antimicrobials in swine production and the appearance of MRSA in humans. MRSA-398 in humans is an infection that originates from swine that were given antimicrobials (often tetracycline). It is difficult, however, to fully demonstrate that antimicrobial consumption in a swine farm had led directly to increased AMR in the human population. The path by which such resistance develops is very complex. Scientific uncertainty will often lead to political uncertainty, such that scientific uncertainty can be transformed into political controversies (Arnoldi 2009).

1.2.2 Governmentality, Risk, and AMR

Michel Foucault has also contributed to the analysis of risks in modern societies. His take on risks is more within the overall framework of 'social construction' (Arnoldi 2009; Bengtsson et al. 2015). Using Foucault's work, it can be argued that risks are nothing in itself. Risks are always part of a social construction where conceptions of risks and non-risks are produced and defined through specific discourses.

The Foucauldian understanding of risk is linked to his concept of governmentality (Foucault 1979, 1991). The concept of governmentality focuses on how the overall nature of government changed in the mid-eighteenth century and how new forms of control developed in the context of the modern state. Modern forms of governmentality are based much less on repression and more on self-regulation among the citizens. Hence, citizens shall take responsibility for themselves and act in accordance with guidelines developed by the state. Often this process is described as a process of subjectivization. Citizens are constructed as subjects.

In the governmentality literature, it is a general observation that the overall governmental structures in late modern societies have changed during the last 30 years. The subjectivization of the citizens has been intensified within a number of policy fields. This has been connected to the neoliberal trends that have gained ground since the 1980s and to overall tendencies towards individualisation. In principle, the process of subjectivization relates to overall questions about how governance is managed and executed. Governance through subjectivization implies that it is the individual citizen who has the responsibility for acting in accordance with the goals stipulated.

In connection with the analysis of risks, the idea of a dominating governmental regime implies that management through self-control becomes a way of structuring risk management. Taking Denmark as an example, regulating the field of antimicrobial consumption through subjectivization is visible in a number of different areas. Hence, patients, livestock farmers, general practitioners, and veterinarians are exposed to a process of subjectivization with respect to their prescription or consumption of antimicrobials.

In Denmark, a number of campaigns against antimicrobials target the general public (particularly patients or potential patients). Patients are informed that antimicrobials shall not be used in a number of situations, especially when they have a virus infection, and patients are expected to refrain from making such demands when they visit their general practitioner. Using Foucault's work, one can say that patients are asked to be subjects in rejecting the use of antimicrobials. Patients are expected to reflect on their own consumption of antimicrobials and then moderate or reject their consumption due to the risks of becoming AMR.

In a parallel way, livestock farmers are also experiencing a process of subjectivization in relation to their use of antimicrobials in the production process. In Denmark, consumption of antimicrobials per animal is measured in every farm and then compared to the average consumption of antimicrobials per animal in Denmark. If a given farmer uses more than the average amount of antimicrobials in their animal production, he or she will be expected to reduce the amount used.

Prescription data for antimicrobials are monitored very specifically with regards to veterinarians in Denmark. The overall amount of prescribed antimicrobials is calculated for every individual veterinarian. If a veterinarian prescribes antimicrobials well beyond the average level of prescription among other veterinarians, they will be asked to explain why they have a higher level of prescription than other veterinarians.

It is noteworthy that the monitoring of consumption of antimicrobials and use of statistics are key mechanisms for controlling antimicrobial consumption and the development of AMR in Denmark. Since the nineteenth century, the use of statistics and measurement has been a major instrument for regimes of governance in the modern state. As Arnoldi observes:

> Knowledge and information about the population are crucial to responsible governments. For that reason, the new technologies that became available in the nineteenth century have played a pivotal role in modern government. It is in fact only by means of statistics that the population can be monitored and hence rendered governable. Data on rates of birth and

> death, health and hygiene, education and skills, work, income, housing, and families are the basis for governing. Such data simply construct, or objectify, the population as a governable object. (Arnoldi 2009, p. 54)

Risks are identified through science and scientific discourses, and risks are the starting point for governmental initiatives. Statistics are the means through which the risks related to specific types of social action (e.g. consumption of antimicrobials) are transformed into governmental objects. This process makes it possible to identify what practices should be governed and how they should be governed.

The fact that statistics are a prerequisite for governance within the field of antimicrobial consumption and AMR is also visible in the various international fora that have discussed antimicrobial consumption and AMR. Due to the global character of AMR, international policy-making organizations such as the EU or UN have initiated action plans intended to reduce the spread of AMR (European Commission 2011; World Health Organization 2014b). In these initiatives, developing statistics about antimicrobial consumption and AMR are crucial for developing and monitoring governmental capacities among the international organizations. The EU, for example, has taken the lead in establishing agencies that monitor antimicrobial consumption and AMR internationally.

As discussed in the former section, risks are identified largely through science and scientific discourses. However, science may also be uncertain about identifying or assessing certain risks. Risks may be identified only as likelihoods or probabilities, in the sense that it becomes likely that this or that type of social action will lead to this or that type of risks. This level of uncertainty is visible, for example, in scientific debates about climate change (Beck 2009).

How societies handle risks is often discussed by using the concept of 'risk management'. Risk management of AMR relates to situations where there is scientific uncertainty. It is possible to identify two types of risk management (Arnoldi 2009, p. 94). In one type, there is a demand for proof of the causality between A and B. One can argue for a ban on A only if it is clearly shown that A is harmful to B. In the second type of risk management, proof is demanded for the non-causality between A and B. Only if it is proven that A is not harmful to B will the use of A be allowed. In the second case, the burden of proof is reversed. This type of risk management is based on the 'principle of uncertainty'. If we take consumption of antimicrobials as an example, we can describe how the two types of risk management could influence how antimicrobials are used.

Among veterinarians, physicians, and microbiologists, there is increasing concern about possible connections between the use of antimicrobials in companion animals and the spread of AMR among the owners of companion animals. This is an important issue because companion animals are sometimes given antimicrobials considered 'critical antimicrobials' (i.e. types of antimicrobials that can be used on humans who show AMR when they receive more ordinary types of antimicrobials). It is also important because we can often observe close physical contact between the companion animals and their owners. The close physical contact is assumed to increase the risks of humans acquiring AMR by their companion animals.

If we apply the first type of risk management to the above-mentioned example, it could be argued that we should not prohibit the use of antimicrobial on companion animals unless we have clear evidence showing a causal link between 'giving the companion animal antimicrobials' and the 'spread of AMR to the owner'. If we apply the 'principle of uncertainty', it could be argued that unless it can be proven that there is no causality between 'giving the companion animal antimicrobials' and 'spread of AMR to the owner', then giving antimicrobials to the companion animals should be restricted or banned.

Risk management is also an activity carried out by 'ordinary' people. They try to perceive the risks that 'escape perception' and try to 'translate' the information they receive from expert communities about these risks into their daily lives and their daily practices. They look for signs that confirm the risks about which they have been informed by the expert communities, and they use these signs as confirmation of the risks, or as evidence that the risk is even greater or lesser than the experts assert. A hot summer, a cold winter, and a windy autumn, for example, can all be interpreted as vagaries of the weather by some people, or as confirmation of irreversible climate change by others.

As part of their interpretative practice, humans also often try to transform the conception of risks into different types of social action. They interpret the risks on the basis of their daily experience and develop social practices that they think can reduce the risks. Some start bicycling instead of driving in their car because they hope that it will help reduce climate change problems. Some participate in social movements in order to change the behaviour of others because they perceive that it is the behaviour of 'the others' that causes climate change problems. Some avoid shaking hands with swine farmers in order to avoid what they perceive as risks of being infected with MRSA.

The interpretation of these types of risks that 'escape perception' does not take place in a social vacuum. On the contrary, the interpretive practices are embedded in existing social structures and in existing types of social differentiation. For a specific group, certain types of social behaviour are thus viewed as normatively acceptable for some social groups, while other types of actions are interpreted as unacceptable. In other social groups, the opposite might be that case. Middle-class people might choose to consume ecological foods as a way of handling risks connected with farmers' use of pesticides, climate change, and AMR. In other social groups, buying ecological food is not at all interpreted as having anything to do with the risks developed in the late modern society.

Both the macro-oriented tendencies in Beck's analysis of the risk society and the more micro-oriented, Foucault-inspired concept of governmentality are highly relevant for the analysis of AMR, its societal embeddedness and its impact. Both perspectives contribute to the understanding of how the risks of AMR—risks that in Beck's terms 'escape perceptions'—have taken a place on the political and scientific agenda in the twenty-first century.

1.3 Presentation of Chapters

This book contains 12 chapters (including this chapter) that elucidate the problem of antimicrobial resistance from various social science/humanistic perspectives.

Some scholars suggest that the authority of Western medical doctors has been in decline for a long time and that patients are becoming increasingly demanding and consumerist. In this light, Beck Nielsen (Chap. 2) presents a single-case analysis of a situation that is particularly interesting: how general practitioners can deal with 'demanding patients' who have their minds set upon antibiotic treatment. These patients come to the consultation requesting penicillin, but they are uninformed of the limitations and potential flipside of the 'miracle drug'. In this situation, doctors may need to adjust patients' expectations and perhaps educate them about appropriate uses of antibiotics. How exactly is such re-adjustment accomplished? Chapter 2 shows in detail how a doctor exploits conversational structures in ways that enables her to avoid a flat-out rejection of the patient's request, turning the situation into one where the patient is informed of the difference between viral and bacterial infections and the dangers of unnecessary use of antibiotics. The key component in the gradual trajectory from responding to the patient's initial request to educating him about the risks of excessive use of antibiotics is the doctor's deferral of stance. The overall lesson from Chap. 2 is that doctors have conversational recourses by which they can deal with demanding patients' requests for antibiotics in responsible ways.

European countries differ substantially both in terms of how much antibiotics their populations consume and in their levels of antimicrobial resistance. With this point of departure, Kragh and Strudsholm (Chap. 3) hypothesize that these differences could be culture-bound, and that such cultural differences could be identified in language use. Kragh and Strudsholm provide a comparative linguistic study of the annual *European Antibiotic Awareness Day* campaign materials targeted at prescribers and potential users in three different language communities: Denmark, France, and Italy. They investigate whether these materials represent different approaches that vary in terms of inclination to choose antibiotic treatment. Could possible differences reflect even further variation in attitudes towards health care and towards the doctor–patient relationship? Sociological research suggests that the Nordic countries may be low-power-distance communities, where doctors and patients act towards each other as social equals. Latin countries (e.g. France and Italy), on the other hand, are generally considered high-power-distance communities, where the hierarchic distance between doctors and patients is great. The comparative study of the campaign materials reveals distinct differences in formality (e.g. infinitive and subjunctive verb formats in French versus use of imperatives in Danish). On the surface, the content aimed at possible prescribers appears similar. But scrutinizing the details, Kragh and Strudsholm observe noteworthy variations: for example, the Danish use of imperatives addresses the potential prescriber directly, while the French and Italian texts are more formal, with indirect use of infinitives. Similarly, the information conveyed to Danish patients/consumers is presented much more directly than its French and Italian counterparts. Altogether, Kragh and Strudsholm's observations point to a more direct form of communication in Denmark, which could indicate a more egalitarian doctor–patient relationship that provides better conditions for lower antibiotic consumption and, thereby, less antimicrobial resistance.

Lindell (Chap. 4) returns to the subject of talk between general practitioners and patients in Denmark and how this talk affects whether or not patients are prescribed antibiotics. Her point of departure is the finding that cough is one of the most common symptoms behind prescribing antibiotics in general practice, and even more important: since the infections that make patients cough tend to be viral rather than bacterial, most of the antibiotic prescriptions are totally ineffective for the individual patient. Instead, they pose a great risk for public health. Lindell's study examines cases where patients complain about persistent cough (i.e. acute bronchitis). Chapter 4 reveals one possible reason why talk about cough can lead to unnecessary prescriptions, and what doctors can do to prevent this. Patients typically introduce the annoying cough in their problem presentation, which is followed by history-taking, examination, and the physician's assessment that the diagnosis is 'merely' a cold and that the patient should wait and see how it develops. However, this message may prompt patients to return to the issue of the persistent cough, which could be interpreted as resistance to the diagnosis and a request/negotiation to receive antibiotic treatment, a situation that is particularly crucial in terms of prescription. Doctors, however, need not automatically assume that patients are reintroducing their symptoms simply because they hope to receive antibiotics. Lindell suggests that this is rarely the reason. Instead of interpreting the re-introduction of cough as an implicit request for antibiotics, how should doctors respond to such concerns? Lindell finds that if doctors re-engage with a symptom presentation and tailor the response to the lifeworld concerns of the patient, not only to a medical ruling out of antibiotics or antibiotic implicative diagnosis (though they also do this), the patients can become reassured and the consultation can be brought to a close. Thus, Lindell's analysis shows that it is indeed possible for doctors to assure patients at these moments without succumbing to the 'solution' by offering a prescription.

De Oliveira, Hernández-Flores, and Rodríguez-Tembras (Chap. 5) point our attention to Spain—and for good reason. Spain is one of the largest consumers of antibiotics for humans in Europe, due partly to the higher frequency of self-medication in Spain. The high level of self-medication is probably a consequence of easier access to antibiotics, which can be purchased at a local pharmacy without prescription. This makes it particularly interesting to examine Spanish prescription practices compared to those of Denmark, which is the purpose of Chap. 5. The authors' study builds upon extensive fieldwork in a rural part of Spain and seeks to provide contextual knowledge about the decision-making process that physicians use to prescribe or not prescribe antibiotics. Analysing their interviews with 24 physicians (general practitioners and geriatric doctors) their data show that physicians clearly recognize the problem of overuse and are aware of the risks involved. So why this excessive use then? General practitioners cite factors such as time management concerns, communication difficulties, patient pressure, proximity difficulties (e.g. patients who live far from the clinic and cannot return for a follow-up), that patients can obtain antibiotics without their assistance anyhow, and so on. Geriatric doctors also acknowledged excessive use of antibiotics within their field, and they attributed the overuse to several factors: severity of geriatrics patients' illnesses and the potential life-threatening risks they entail, the risk of prolonged hospitalization without antibiotic treatment, the preventive benefits of using antibiotics in geriatrics, and so on. Chapter 5 contributes to the understanding of overuse of antibiotics by mapping Spanish professionals' explanations for their prescribing practices. This can form the basis for future research and for productive dialogues between professionals and policy makers.

Jensen (Chap. 6) presents various national government structures and regulative frameworks, as well as the WHO's international initiatives towards current and future risks of human health related to antimicrobial resistance. In this context, Jensen analyses how those structures and frameworks influence the use of antibiotics in different countries. The interrelationship between the use of antibiotics and different types of resistance towards the rules differs from one country to another, an indication that national attempts at governing the use of antibiotics, for example, in order to prevent further proliferation of antimicrobial resistance, cause different types of resistance among local farmers. Chapter 6 then zooms in on Denmark as an interesting case for two reasons: Denmark's relatively strong regulations and governance both in the human and the veterinarian sectors and a relatively low use of antibiotics among both humans and animals. Finally, Jensen discusses current challenges for the possible alignment of stronger governance in other countries.

In Chap. 7, Fynbo moves the macro perspective of Chap. 6 to a much narrower and micro-oriented discussion of how Danish farmers control the lives of pigs via antibiotics. Chapter 7 takes the reader on a tour of large Danish pig farms, introducing us to the lives of the pigs: how are they treated during their different life stages, how the pig farmers control the pigs' lives, and what kind of knowledge is activated through this type of production? The pigs, it is argued, are temporal constructions of life, dependent on the farmers and how and when the farmers decide to use antibiotics as a central means of controlling the pigs' lives. Chapter 7 uses an actor–network perspective and a combination of qualitative interviews with farmers and veterinarians and field studies of several pig farms.

Chapter 8 (Jensen and Fynbo) studies how the outspoken criticism of Danish pig production leads to social stigmatization of people in the pig industry, including pig farmers and their families. In Denmark, as well as in most other Western countries, the emergence of MRSA has led to considerable criticism of pig producers and their perceived neglect of public health. Nevertheless, the actual number of human MRSA cases is still relatively small in Denmark, with an average of just one MRSA case per year. On the other hand, national statistics show a relatively strong rise in human MRSA infections. Chapter 8 does not delve deeper into the extent of risk caused by Danish pig producers to public health. Based on qualitative interviews with pig farmers, scientific experts, and other stakeholders, Jensen and Fynbo instead describe how expert knowledge about antimicrobial resistance sometimes generates very sceptical public opinions and how those opinions are experienced as stigmatization by the pig farmers. By differentiating between three types of stigmatization, Chap. 8 shows how the pig farmers tend to accept the special attention and risk management that they receive at hospitals and in the health sector, as long as those special measures are based on scientific knowledge and risk analysis. However, Jensen and Fynbo also show how the pig farmers struggle with overcoming the negative image that they have obtained through some of the very outspoken scientific experts. The pig farmers' feelings of stigmatization can become a barrier for their efforts to manage their pigs without the use of antibiotics.

In a similar vein, Pedersen and Jepsen (Chap. 9) focus on good doctoring in times where antimicrobial resistance is conceived as a global threat to public health. In such risky circumstances, doctors' decision-making is a complex issue: if they prescribe too much antibiotics, they not only risk public health at national as well as international level, they also risk losing effective antibiotics, which has been one of their most valued tools in clinical practice since the mid-1950s. Pedersen and Jepsen apply a professions perspective to study a number of recordings of consultations between GPs and patients aimed at acquiring antibiotics for colds and infections: how do professional medical practitioners govern and control prescribing antibiotics in a Danish primary care setting? And how do contemporary notions of good doctoring influence the doctors handling and care of their patients? Drawing on abductive analysis, Pedersen and Jepsen find that along with their technical expertise, the doctors' informal knowledge and clinical etiquette are also essential factors contributing to good doctoring.

Bank and Rogne (Chap. 10) study how Danish general practitioners manage uncertainty related to when and how to prescribe antibiotics. Modern-day GPs not only have to manage their own uncertainty about the public health risks related to prescribing antibiotics (similar to the uncertainties of pig farmers). They also often have to relate their own uncertainty to the affective states of their patients, and they must do so in the special setting of the clinical encounter. In a combined actor–network and governmentality perspective and based on qualitative data from consultation sessions between GPs and patients, Bank and Rogne analyse how the primary task of contemporary GPs in a modern welfare state such as Denmark is not that of diagnosing and prescribing but rather, of managing how knowledge, communication, bodily states, and affectivity affect the clinical encounter between GP and patient. Bank and Rogne define this ability as a 'psy-medical competence' activated in the 'no-treatment' part of the consultation. Sometimes, the GPs use their psy-medical competence to turn complex medical discourse into common talk, a transformation that may indeed help patients overcome their own uncertainty. Sometimes, the GPs deploy their psy-medical competences more explicitly towards governing patients' affective states, while on other occasions their psy-medical competence enables the GPs to simply perform good doctoring. Bank and Rogne challenge the notion of doctoring as an objective, techno-scientific skill. Chapter 10 concludes that contemporary GPs depend on their psy-medical competence to bridge the gaps between issues of knowledge, materiality and psycho-social questions.

Chapter 11 (Jepsen and Pedersen) focuses on antimicrobial resistance as a global problem. The contributions of this volume make it clear that the use of antibiotics has created a risky paradox: the continuous application of antibiotics is likely to cause more antimicrobial resistance. In relation to treating microbial infections, the modern world has reached a cul-de-sac. We now have to find new technical solutions in treating both humans and animals. Furthermore, while still lacking new therapeutic agents in the pharmaceutical pipelines, the entire world is at risk. There is a major need to develop new policies and programmes of surveillance and governance in order to advance more prudent use amongst professionals. Chapter 11 focuses on the social ecology comprised by the paradoxical interrelationship between antibiotics as a common good threatened by antimicrobial resistance, but which is itself caused by the use of these same antibiotics. If there ever was an archetypal 'vicious circle', this is one.

In this book's final chapter, Jensen, Nielsen, and Fynbo summarize the results of the research presented in the chapters. We also comment on the new global political initiatives regarding AMR, underscoring the crucial need for a broader social science perspective in the struggle against AMR.

References

Arnoldi, J. (2009). *Risk: An introduction*. Cambridge: Polity Press.

Beck, U. (1992). *Risk society: Towards a new modernity, theory, culture & society*. London and Newbury Park, CA: Sage Publications.

Beck, U. (2009). *World at risk*. Cambridge: Polity Press.

Bengtsson, T. T., Frederiksen, M., & Larsen, J. E. (2015). Is risk transforming the Danish welfare state? In *The Danish welfare state: A sociological investigation* (pp. 3–21). New York, Houndmills, Basingstoke: Palgrave Macmillan.

Bonilla, A. R., & Muniz, K. P. (Eds.). (2009). *Antibiotic resistance: Causes and risk factors, mechanisms and alternatives, pharmacology: Research, safety testing and regulation series*. New York: Nova Science Publishers.

Drlica, K., & Perlin, D. (2011). *Antibiotic resistance: Understanding and responding to an emerging crisis*. Upper Saddle River, NJ: FT Press.

European Commission. (2011). Communication from the Commission to the European Parliament and the Council—Action plan against the rising threats from antimicrobial resistance. European Commission, Com 748.

European Commission. (2015). ECDC/EFSA/EMA first joint report on the integrated analysis of the consumption of antimicrobial agents and occurrence of antimicrobial resistance in bacteria from humans and food-producing animals. Europeam Food Safety Authority.

Foucault, M. (1979). On governmentality. *Ideology & Consciousness, 6*, 5–21.

Foucault, M. (1991). Governmentality. In G. Burchell, C. Gordon, & P. Miller (Eds.), *The Foucault effect: Studies in governmentality* (pp. 87–105). Chicago: University of Chicago Press.

Podolsky, S. H. (2006). *Pneumonia before antibiotics: Therapeutic evolution and evaluation in twentieth-century America*. Baltimore, MD: Johns Hopkins University Press.

Podolsky, S. H. (2015). *The antibiotic era: Reform, resistance, and the pursuit of a rational therapeutics*. Baltimore, MD: Johns Hopkins University Press.

Stivers, T. (2007). *Prescribing under pressure: Parent-physician conversations and antibiotics*. Oxford: Oxford University Press.

World Health Organization (Ed.). (2014a). *Antimicrobial resistance: Global report on surveillance*. Geneva: World Health Organization.

World Health Organization (Ed.). (2014b). *Antimicrobial resistance: Global report on surveillance*. Geneva: World Health Organization.

World Health Organization. (2015). *Worldwide country situation analysis: Response to antimicrobial resistance*. Geneva: WHO.

2

Dealing with Explicit Patient Demands for Antibiotics in a Clinical Setting

Søren Beck Nielsen

2.1 Introduction

This chapter focusses on language use in authentic general practice consultations. There are two reasons why this topic is worthy of inquiry. First, general practice plays an essential role in the Danish health care system, where general practitioners act as gatekeepers to various medical services, including issuing prescriptions (see Beck Nielsen 2011; Pedersen et al. 2012). Consequently, approximately 90% of the antimicrobial human consumption stems from primary health care (see Danmap 2014, p. 17). However, antibiotic resistance is currently a much bigger problem in the hospital sector, and recent research suggests that potentially inappropriate use under the auspices of primary care can be a direct cause of high levels of antibiotic resistance (Costelloe et al. 2014). It is therefore very important to understand how potentially inappropriate antibiotics

S. B. Nielsen (✉)
Department of Nordic Studies and Linguistics, University of Copenhagen, Copenhagen, Denmark
e-mail: sbnielsen@hum.ku.dk

C. S. Jensen et al. (eds.), *Risking Antimicrobial Resistance*,
https://doi.org/10.1007/978-3-319-90656-0_2

are prescribed as part of primary care and how doctors can avoid overprescribing.

For the past 20 years, Danish officials have monitored the consumption of antibiotics among humans and animals and published the results in the annual Danish Integrated Antimicrobial Resistance Monitoring and Research Programme (DANMAP) reports. The results show a worrying general increase in antimicrobial resistance. One of the latest reports speculates why: 'It is assumed that patient demands for receiving antibiotic treatment may play an important role in the increasing total consumption of antimicrobial drugs as well as causing changes observed in the consumption of individual antimicrobial agents' (Danmap 2015, p. 49).

This hypothesis brings us to this chapter's second raison d'être: the role of the language used that leads to or does not lead to patients being prescribed antibiotics when they visit their family doctor. Language pervades all aspects, phases, and activities of clinical encounters, regardless of whether doctors base their diagnosis upon talks alone (i.e. patient's explanations and the discussions they lead to) or an oral consultation supported by more objective diagnostic means such as point of care tests or unmediated diagnostic measures such as physically inspecting patients' bodily symptoms (Heritage et al. 2010).

A considerable amount of research has been devoted to mapping the ways in which language use effects diagnoses, treatment recommendations, and possibly antibiotic prescriptions. This chapter contributes to this line of research with a conversation analytic single-case analysis of a scenario that has not yet been addressed from a discursive point of view. Using a video-recorded Danish consultation where a patient explicitly asks for penicillin we examine how doctors deal with overt demands for antibiotics. The combination of patients thinking that they know what they need and their demand for medication may be a scenario that doctors will experience more frequently in the future. As such, patients will increasingly inform themselves about the internet before visiting their doctor (e.g. Caiata-Zufferey and Schulz 2012). This scenario could be considered an extreme variant of the aforementioned hypothesis regarding 'patient demands for receiving antibiotic treatment'. It differs markedly from patients' more subtle tactics of insisting on antibiotics as their appropriate treatment plan, which have been extensively explored in previous research—as the next section will show.

2.2 Expressions of Treatment Expectations in the Clinic

According to language philosopher M. M. Bakhtin, there 'can be no such thing as an absolutely neutral utterance' (1986, p. 84). That is, speakers always express a stance towards any given topic, and, importantly, listeners inherently look for a stance. Bakhtin's reminder is appropriate in our context. Naturally, patients' symptoms may be described in more neutral terms with respect to whether or not they should be treated with antibiotics. According to Bakhtin, however, doctors might easily perceive patients' neutral descriptions as ways of 'fishing' for offers to receive antibiotic treatment.

Several studies have documented a persistent connection between doctors' perceptions of patients' expectations towards antibiotic treatment and their prescription practices: if doctors sense that patients expect antibiotics, they are more prone to prescribe them (Britten and Ukoumunne 1997; Mangione-Smith et al. 2004; Stivers et al. 2003). This association may have something to do with doctors' wishes to obtain patient satisfaction. Recent studies reveal that antibiotic prescription volume is highly correlated with patient satisfaction in the UK (e.g. Ashworth et al. 2016), and doctors can successfully utilize certain protocols for treatment recommendations in order to improve their ratings (Mangione Smith et al. 2015). However, doctors surely risk overestimating patients' expectations of receiving antibiotic treatment—as suggested by a recent British interview study (Mustafa et al. 2014) and an American survey study in paediatrics that compared parents' pre-consultation expectations of possible antibiotic treatment with doctors' post-consultation perceptions of parents' expectations (Mangione-Smith et al. 2004).

Some scholars have examined which patterns of communicative behaviour enhance doctors' assumptions of patients' expectations regarding antibiotic treatment. An American survey study suggests that doctors are most likely to assume that patients expect antibiotic treatment when patients convey resistance to doctors' deliveries of viral diagnoses (Stivers et al. 2003). However, doctors are likely to react to many other and much more subtle cues. Tanya Stivers' (2007), in her pioneering work on implicit ways of negotiating antibiotic treatment in American paediatric consultations, finds that parents put doctors under pressure to prescribe antibiotics regularly, though not necessarily consciously. For example, parents can foreground the relevance of antibiotics in problem presentations (e.g. proposing infections as candidate diagnoses), they can respond to illness history questions in ways that challenge their treatment implications, they can resist diagnoses (e.g. via questioning the doctor), and they can resist treatment recommendations (e.g. via refusal to accept a prescription or treatment regime).

Thus, research provides us detailed information about the kind of treatment-related negotiations that takes place at an implicit level, that is, without patients asking explicitly for antibiotics. We know considerably less about what happens when patients explicitly request antibiotics from their doctors. This is perhaps because explicit requests seem to occur quite infrequently. A British observational study of 29 sore throat consultations, for example, report of no occurrences where patients explicitly requested antibiotics (Rollnick et al. 2001). Furthermore, patients' explicit insistence on antibiotic treatment may exhibit fewer regularities in terms of sequential positioning: Stivers (2007, p. 131) remarks that 'overt lobbying for antibiotics occurs in virtually all phases of the medical encounter'. The overt cases cited by Stivers are those she categorizes as requests for antibiotics, stating a desire for antibiotics, inquiring about antibiotics, and mentions of past experience with antibiotic treatment. The common feature of these more overt requests is that patients explicitly utter the word 'antibiotics'. However, there may be significant differences between, for example, hinting that a condition could be cured with the help of antibiotics by mentioning past experiences and directly requesting them. One important difference lies in how the doctor might respond, ranging from acceding to the request to rejecting it. The question here, however, is whether Stivers' data fully allow us for such an assessment. She finds only two cases of outright requests for antibiotics, and the example she examines is a case where a parent, following a wait-and-see diagnosis as a 'last resort', asks a doctor: 'Can I at least have the prescription, and I'll decide whether or not to fill it in a couple of days?' (p. 138). Thus, the parent's insistence, Stivers concludes, is 'an intrusion into the physician's domain of expertise' (p. 137).

In this chapter, I analyse a conversation based on a similar overt request for antibiotics. This particular patient constructs his request for antibiotics in a less mitigated manner and not as a 'last resort'. In fact, obtaining antibiotics is presented as the main reason for the patient's visit. This behaviour fits well with some of the core characteristics that reflect a trend towards patient consumerism (e.g. Timmermans and Oh 2010). One of the positive aspects of patients taking on a more assertive consumer role is that patients actively participate in decision-making processes. One of the negative aspects, however, is that these engaged patients may have decided in advance what they suffer from and how they should be treated. This kind of assertive consumerism can undermine the diagnostic procedure. Gill (2005, p. 470) therefore recommends that 'In this era of relatively well-informed patients and various (and at times conflicting) imperatives for physicians, it is important to understand how patients advocate for their own health care and how physicians respond'. This chapter, taking its point of departure in this advice, examines a similar kind of interaction and the effects on how antibiotics are prescribed.

2.3 Data and Method

The analysis is based on a video-recorded consultation, recorded over the winter months of 2008–2009 at a large general practice clinic in a large Danish town. The consultation was recorded with the informed approval and written consent of both doctor and patient. The example is selected from a corpus of 52 recordings as the one most strongly representing an overt request of antibiotics.

Conversation analysis is a scientific approach that originated in the early 1960s and unites elements of sociology and linguistics. It is used to investigate the organization of talk-in-interaction. Conversation analysts pay close attention not only to *what* people say, but to *how* and *when* they say what they do. The conversation analytic approach thus involves a rigorous inspection of the situated linguistic and embodied means by which actors jointly seek to establish shared understanding. Hence, conversation analytical transcripts also include paralinguistic details such as stress, prolongations, intonation, prosody, and overlapping talk (see the appended list of notation symbols). The Danish transcription is presented in italics above the aligned English translation.

The following presents a single-case analysis—as opposed to an examination of a conglomeration of related occurrences, which of course precludes any kind of generalizability. However, single-case analyses are valuable because they allow for the exploration of rich details of 'uncharted territory' (Schegloff 1993). In this particular case, the territory to be explored is how doctors deal with patients' explicit demands for antibiotics.

2.4 Analysis

The doctor, an experienced female general practitioner, is abbreviated as DOC. The patient, a male in his early forties, is abbreviated as PAT. This following exchange occurs at the beginning of the consultation:

(Ex 1): 0:05-0:49

```
01. DOC: Hej.
         Hello.

02. PAT: Altså- jeg tænkte bare på om jeg ikke kunne få noget penicillin
         You know- I merely wondered if I could have some penicillin

03.      til øh min ↑hals, .hh
         for erh my throat, .hh

04. DOC: ↑Ja.
          Yes.

05. PAT: Fordi lige om lidt så har jeg så dårlig hals øh så nu må jeg
         Because very shortly I'll have such a bad throat erh that I'd

06.      hellere tage det i opløbet og jeg har simpelthen så meget arbejde.
         better nip it in the bud and I just have so much work to do.

07.      .hhhh *<Så ø:hm> jeg skal lave ((arbejde)) på fredag og puh .h
         .hhhh  <So erhm> I'm doing ((work)) on Friday and phew .h
               *DO nods her head vertically

08. PAT: Og jeg gider bare ikke have halsbetændelse. Og det får jeg

         And I just don't want to suffer from a throat infection. And I
         will get it

09.      lige om lidt jeg har det NÆSTEN. ((synker)) ø::hm Og så
         in a minute. I ALMOST have it. ((swallows)) e:rhm And so

10.      tænkte jeg ba(h)re med hi:t med noget penici[llin. heh heh
         I ju(h)st thought gimme some                 penicillin. hah ha
```

11. DOC: [((laughs))

12. PAT: *Jeg har prøvet det så mange gange før* [*så jeg ved præcis*
I've tried it so many times before so I know exactly
13. DOC: [**Har du det?*
Have you?
*DO quickly gazes at her computer screen
14. PAT: *hvad det handler om.*
what it's about.

15. DOC: °*Ja*°.
Yes.

16. (.)

17. DOC: *Får du- har du altid bak↑terier når du har halsbetændelse*?
Do you- is it always bacterial when you get a sore throat?

18. PAT: *Ja.*
Yes.

19. (.7)

20. PAT: *Ja eller det ved jeg ikke hvad sp- hvad spørgsmål det forstår jeg ikke.*
Yes or I don't know what that ques- that question I don't understand.

21. DOC: *.hh De:t fordi °a:t° h. langt over halvdelen af de halsbetændelser*
.hh It's because .h far more than half of the sore throats

22. *vi får de skyldes virus.*
we get are caused by viruses.

23. PAT: *Okay.*
Okay.

24. DOC: *Og derfor laver vi altid en test hernede for ikke a:t sprøjte om os*
And that's why we always do a test down here not to give

25. *med penicillin som ikke gavner.*
penicillin injections left right and centre that don't do any good.

26. PAT: *Okay.*
Okay.

27. DOC: *Så jeg vil gerne ↑teste dig* (...)
So I'd like to test you (...)

28. (.3)

28. PAT: *Okay °men° det må du godt* (...)
Okay, but you can do that (...)

In line 02–03, the patient asks for a penicillin prescription for his sore throat. He persistently explains why he should receive a prescription, explicitly pressuring the doctor's assessment. Gail Jefferson (1984) has noted that speakers can move away from talking about troublesome matters to more light-hearted issues in stepwise manners. A similar process is observed here. The doctor's methodical use of a list of conversational resources in response to the patient's request and subsequent actions enables her to convert the situation to one where she is the expert educating the patient about why his initial expectations may not be correct, and that he just might not need antibiotics after all.

The first systematic resource is to defer the stance towards the patient's request by passing the floor on several possible occasions. The patient introduces his request with a distancing 'I wondered if'-clause (Fox and Heinemann 2016). However, the subsequent request for penicillin is formulated with negative polarity, whereby the patient displays a relatively high level of entitlement, that is, anticipates acceptance. The request proper is completed with the specifying prepositional phrase 'for my throat'. The doctor could then relevantly express her stance towards the request. But she could also treat the patient's steady prosody and in-breath as displays of having more talk to add. By 'merely' uttering an intonationally rising yes-token in line 04, the doctor elects the latter option.

The next occasion where the doctor might express her stance takes place after the first possible completed part of the patient's account for why he requests penicillin in line 06, where the patient announces, with epistemic certainty, that he is developing a sore throat and asserts that it can and should be 'nipped in the bud' with penicillin. The patient hints that it will otherwise interfere with his work load. Again, the doctor simply encourages the patient to continue instead of answering 'yes' or 'no', this time with a head nod (line 07). The patient treats the encouragement to continue—but perhaps also the lack of affirmation—as an incentive to push his argumentation. He pressures the doctor even further. Firstly, he specifies the work task (deleted for the sake of anonymity) that is threatened by his sore throat. Second, the patient expresses reluctance about suffering from the condition ('I just don't want'). Third, the patient refers to his condition in line 08 with the clinical term a 'throat infection'

(Danish: *halsbetændelse*) as opposed to the previous vernacular reference 'bad throat' (Danish: *dårlig hals*) in line 05. Fourth, by epistemically upgrading the assertion that this condition is imminent ('I will in a minute, I almost do'), which—supported by the projection of direct reported speech ('and so I just thought')—paves the way for what could be interpreted by the physician as a demand for penicillin in line 10. This apparent demand is designed as a strong imperative: 'gimme some penicillin'. But the doctor laughs at this demand in line 11.

Laughter thus makes up the doctor's second systematic resource. By laughing, the doctor continues to defer the stance towards the patient's request, and she indicates that the patient's strong imperative is not to be taken seriously. At first sight, the doctor begins to laugh *before* the patient himself bursts out. On closer inspection, however, we see that the patient actually anticipates the initial signs of laughability already in the aspiration that accompanies the vowel in the word 'bare' (English: just) in line 10. Thus, the doctor may in fact be laughing *with* instead of laughing *at* here (see Glenn 2003, Chaps. 4 and 5). Another factor that enables the doctor to further defer her stance towards the patient's request is that the strong imperative in line 10 is produced as reported speech using a projecting verb in past tense (i.e. 'thought'). That is, the patient's imperative can therefore be interpreted by the physician not only as a momentary demand but also—and perhaps more—as an explanation of how he felt earlier, thus accounting for why he has requested penicillin earlier in the exchange.

The doctor's third systematic resource is to defer the decision by inquiring as to the patient's history, in line 17. Again, this move is occasioned by the patient, who draws on his experience with similar conditions in the past (lines 12–14). Furthermore, the inquiry is actively prepared by the doctor herself, as she intervenes in the first part of the patient's expressed reasoning (i.e. 'I've tried it so many times before') and simply replies 'Have you?' while briefly gazing at her computer. The act of posing a question prepares the recipient that the speaker might have more to say after hearing the answer (Sacks 1992, pp. 49–63, 246). In this case, the patient effectively stops talking after the brief confirmative answer in line 15. This particular question's focus also alludes to what the doctor might simultaneously be searching for on the computer screen: checking if the patient has a history of sore throats, which makes an activity transition towards history-taking relevant (Beck Nielsen 2016). Initially treating the medically important distinction between bacterial versus viral conditions as understood, the polar yes/no history-taking question in line 17 seeks to establish whether the patient's recurrent sore throats tend to be caused by bacteria. This is the question's candidate answer, that is, its best guess. Its use of the extreme case formulation 'always' is also worth noting (Pomerantz 1986). Still deferring a stance, the doctor nonetheless remains formally 'friendly' towards the patient's request, account and immediately prior comment that he knows 'exactly what it is about', with these two question design features. Together, they convey that the patient's self-diagnosis might easily be correct, and that the infection could be bacterial this time as well. However, the question also opens the possibility that the patient does not know 'exactly what it is about'. In that case, an educational lesson about the appropriate use of antibiotics could be a relevant conversational turn.

The doctor's fourth and final systematic resource is to wait for the patient to present his affirmative reply (line 18) to the question of whether his history of sore throats usually tend to be bacterial. The affirmative 'yes' is produced without the least hesitation or reservation. Yet the doctor, instead of confirming the patient's reply, remains silent (in line 19). The silence makes the patient resume his 'yes' reply, but immediately afterwards—with an 'or' self-correction—the patient expresses difficulties understanding the question. The doctor uses this display of non-understanding as a stepping stone to explain not only how the question should be understood, but also why it is an important one. Hence, the doctor commences her explanation with 'It's because'. She continues by explaining that more than half the sore throat cases she witnesses are viral; that is, she invokes a statistical fact to account for why her question about the patient's history is paramount. She further supplements the statistical lesson with a procedural one. With the turn-initial 'and therefore', the doctor thus substantiates why she always tests for infections in order not to erroneously 'give up penicillin left right and centre'. In addition to demonstrating her own expertise, the doctor thus also enlightens the patient about proper use of antibiotics, hints at the effects of inappropriate use, and reiterates her initial reluctance to accede to the patient's request.

This example began with a rather blunt request by the patient. It ends with the patient accepting the doctor's offer to undergo a bacteriological test. This option is conveyed as an offer by means of the Danish adverb '*gerne*' that—among others—may have a 'granting' meaning, expressing that an action is done out of courtesy to its recipient (see Hansen and Heltoft 2011, p. 783). Harvey Sacks has proposed that utterances are heard to convey the most there is to say about something. He called this the 'maximal property of descriptions' (Sacks 1992). Sacks' concept is demonstrated in this excerpt, where the doctor—in offering to test the patient—makes it clear that this is the most she is willing to grant the patient at the moment. The patient accepts with an 'Okay', though slightly reluctantly ('but you can do that…')—presumably recognizing that this test is all that he will be offered at the moment. The doctor has thus, successfully managed to refute the patient's expectations regarding a prescription without further diagnostic evidence, and she has done this without overtly dismissing his request.

2.5 Concluding Remarks

It is crucial to reduce the inappropriate use of antibiotics among humans and animals alike in order to successfully combat antimicrobial resistance. Social scientists can help in this effort by identifying the practices that lead to the potentially inappropriate use of antibiotics. Some of these practices are governmental and can be investigated via macro-oriented analyses (Strøby Jensen 2018). Others are interactional and should be examined via detailed micro-oriented analyses. This chapter has contributed to the latter perspective.

As mentioned, it is the Danish Health Authority's hypothesis that patient demands cause the increasing consumption of antibiotics, and that this increased consumption leads to resistance and endangers treatment possibilities. A test of this hypothesis would be a valuable goal to pursue in future research. Such a test could also address the popular assumption—correct or exaggerated—that patients feel more informed about personal health matters because of easily available information online, and that they therefore increasingly participate in treatment decisions in the form of insistence for demands to their doctors. However, it might also be the case that patients may be less informed than they think they are. They may, therefore, insist on inappropriate, if not risky, treatments. In this study, we encountered a patient who was totally convinced of his need for penicillin. However, it turned out that he was unaware—like many of us—of the important distinction between symptoms caused by bacteria and symptoms caused by viruses. The doctor dealt with the patient's misguided request by informing the patient of the difference between bacteria- and virus-based illnesses and of the proper diagnostic procedure.

The occasional need for doctors to educate patients is apparent in this particular case. Generally, such educational efforts are recognized as one of the important ways to reduce inappropriate use of antibiotics and thereby combat antimicrobial resistance. One of the questions raised by this need for better patient education is when to educate patients during consultations. Stivers (2007, p. 191) argues that patients are unreceptive to such education prior to receiving an affirmative, specific, and non-mimimized diagnosis and treatment recommendation. If such educational explanations are given in response to patients' problem presentations, doctors risk treating a symptom's complaint as an implicit request for antibiotics. However, if antibiotics were not what the patient had in mind, the doctor risks making antibiotics into an issue when it need not be. In the case study described here, demanding antibiotics was an overt issue from the outset because of the patient's initial and explicit request. Furthermore, this doctor accompanied the medical explanation of the difference between bacterial and viral infections with a procedural one: patients should be tested positive before they are prescribed antibiotics. These explanations effectively made the patient revise his demand and accept the proper diagnostic procedure. In this case, the argument against a premature educational explanation, therefore, comes across as unpersuasive.

The issue of precisely when it is appropriate for doctors to explain to patients about the difference between a viral and bacterial infection points to the challenge associated with producing general recommendations and guidelines that are supported by rigorous social scientific research. In spite of the fact that medical consultations usually progress in orderly phases, it is very difficult to produce guidelines that can cover every feasible situation in a real-life consultation. As Lucy Suchman (2009, p. 52) succinctly states: 'The coherence of situated action is tied in essential ways not to individual predispositions or conventional rules but to local interactions contingent on the actor's particular circumstances.'

In order to resist patient pressure and avoid prescribing inappropriate antibiotics, doctors thus need to attend carefully to each of the patient's verbal actions, deal with patients' unstated assumptions, and try to steer the interaction in a desirable direction. In the case analysed by her, a doctor successfully managed not only to avoid giving in to the patient's demand, but also to inform him why his demand was misguided. The means by which the doctor succeeded comprised four specific ways of deferring a stance: (1) use of continuer tokens, (2) laughter, (3) history-taking inquiry, and (4) awaiting the patient's own recognition of non-understanding. Each element was produced as a response to the patient's actions, and each element had an impact on how subsequent interaction developed.

Together, the interaction occasioned an opportunity to explain essential diagnostic and procedural principles that could rebut the patient's medically inappropriate expectations. The lessons from this detailed study are that doctors have conversational recourses available to them with which they can deal with patients' demands for antibiotics in responsible ways. With an increasing number of assertive patients who insist that they are well informed, it would be advisable for doctors to undergo more sophisticated 'conversational training' in order to deal with these patients.

Appendix: Transcription Symbols

[	The beginning of overlapping speech
]	The end of overlapping speech
(.)	A pause under 0.2 seconds
(0.5)	A pause measured in seconds
(comment)	Comment about the translation

=	Uttered with no pause at all
:	Prolonged sound
word	Emphatic
WORD	Increased volume
°word°	Soft spoken
<word>	Slow speech
>word<	Fast speech
.h	In-breath
wo(h)rd	Laughing voice
heh heh	laughter
wor-	A cut-off, i.e. a sudden speech stop
XX	Unintelligible
*	Notation of embodied conduct that coincides with speech
↑word	Rising intonation
↓word	Falling intonation
punctuation mark after turn-unit.	Falling prosody
comma after turn-unit,	Steady prosody
question mark after turn-unit?	Rising prosody

References

Ashworth, M., White, P., Jongsma, H., Schofield, P., & Armstrong, D. (2016). Antibiotic prescribing and patient satisfaction in primary care in England: Cross-sectional analysis of national patient survey data and prescribing data. *British Journal of General Practice, 66*(642), e40–e46.

Bakhtin, M. M. (1986). *Speech genres and other late essays*. Austin: University of Texas Press.

Beck Nielsen, S. (2011). Keeping the gate ajar during openings of general practice consultations. *Communication & Medicine, 8*(3), 235–245.

Beck Nielsen, S. (2016). How doctors manage consulting computer records while interacting with patients. *Research on Language and Social Interaction, 41*(1), 58–74.

Britten, N., & Ukoumunne, O. (1997). The influence of patients' hopes of receiving a prescription on doctors' perceptions and the decision to prescribe: A questionnaire survey. *BMJ, 6; 315*(7121), 1506–1510.

Caiata-Zufferey, M., & Schulz, P. J. (2012). Physicians' communicative strategies in interacting with internet-informed patients: Results from a qualitative study. *Health Communication, 27*(8), 738–749.

Costelloe, C., Martin Williams, O., Montgomery, A. A., Dayan, C., & Alastair, H. D. (2014). Antibiotic prescribing in primary care and antimicrobial resistance in patients admitted to hospital with urinary tract infection: A controlled observational pilot study. *Antibiotics, 3*(1), 29–38.

Danmap. (2014). *Use of antimicrobial agents and occurrence of antimicrobial resistance in bacteria from food animals, food and humans in Denmark*. Available from: https://www.danmap.org/Downloads/Reports.aspx

Danmap. (2015). *Use of antimicrobial agents and occurrence of antimicrobial resistance in bacteria from food animals, food and humans in Denmark*. Available from: https://www.danmap.org/Downloads/Reports.aspx

Fox, B., & Heinemann, T. (2016). Rethinking format: An examination of requests. *Language in Society, 45*(4), 499–531.

Gill, V. T. (2005). Patient 'demand' for medical interventions: Exerting pressure for an offer in a primary care clinic visit. *Research on Language and Social Interaction, 38*(4), 451–479.

Glenn, P. (2003). *Laughter in interaction*. Cambridge: Cambridge University Press.

Hansen, E., & Heltoft, L. (2011). *Grammatik over det danske sprog: Syntaktiske og semantiske enheder*. København: Det Danske Sprog- og litteraturselskab.

Heritage, J., Elliott, M., Stivers, T., Richardson, A., & Mangione-Smith, R. (2010). Reducing inappropriate antibiotics prescribing: The role of online commentary on physical examination findings. *Patient Education and Counseling, 81*, 119–125.

Jefferson, G. (1984). On stepwise transition from talk about trouble to inappropriately next-positioned matters. In J. Maxwell & J. Heritage (Eds.), *Structures of social action. Studies in conversation analysis* (pp. 191–222). Cambridge: Cambridge University Press.

Mangione-Smith, R., Elliott, M., Stivers, T., McDonald, L., Heritage, J., & McGlynn, E. A. (2004). Racial/ethnic variation in parent expectations for antibiotics: Implications for public health campaigns. *Pediatrics, 113*(5), e385–e394.

Mangione Smith, R., Zhou, C., Robinson, J. D., Taylor, J. A., Elliott, M. N., & Heritage, J. (2015). Communication practices and antibiotic use for acute respiratory tract infections in children. *Annals of Family Medicine, 13*, 221–227.

Mustafa, M., Wood, F., Butler, C. C., & Elwyn, G. (2014). Managing expectations of antibiotics for upper respiratory tract infections: A qualitative study. *Annals of Family Medicine, 12*(1), 29–36.

Pedersen, K. M., Andersen, J. S., & Søndergaard, J. (2012). General practice and primary health care in Denmark. *Journal of the American Board of Family Medicine, 25*, 34–38.

Pomerantz, A. (1986). Extreme case formulations: A way of legitimizing claims. *Human Studies, 9*(2–3), 219–229.

Rollnick, S., Seale, C., Rees, M., Butler, C., Kinnersley, P., & Anderson, L. (2001). Inside the routine general practice consultation: An observational study of consultations for sore throats. *Family Practice, 18*(5), 506–510.

Sacks, H. (1992). *Lectures on conversation* (Vol. 1). Malden, MA: Blackwell.

Schegloff, E. A. (1993). Reflections on quantification in the study of conversation. *Research on Language and Social Interaction, 26*(1), 99–128.

Stivers, T. (2007). *Prescribing under pressure: Parent-physician conversations and antibiotics*. Oxford: Oxford University Press.

Stivers, T., Mangione-Smith, R., Elliott, M., McDonald, L., & Heritage, J. (2003). Why do physicians think parents expect antibiotics? What parents report vs. what physicians believe. *Journal of Family Practice, 52*(2), 140–148.

Strøby Jensen, C. (2018). Governing the consumption of antimicrobials: The Danish model for using antimicrobials in a comparative perspective. In C. Strøby Jensen, S. B. Nielsen, & L. Fynbo (Eds.), *Risking antimicrobial resistance* (pp. 25–40). Cham, Switzerland: Palgrave Macmillan.

Suchman, L. A. (2009). *Human-machine reconfigurations. Plans and situated actions* (2nd ed.). Cambridge: Cambridge University Press.

Timmermans, S., & Oh, H. (2010). The continued social transformation of the medical profession. The continued social transformation of the medical profession. *Journal of Health and Social Behavior, 51*(S), 94–106.

3

Antibiotics in France and Italy: A Linguistic Analysis of Policies and Practices Compared to Danish Standards

Kirsten A. Jeppesen Kragh and Erling Strudsholm

3.1 Introduction

Taking as a starting point the statistical evidence that antibiotic resistance is greater in Southern than Northern Europe (see e.g. Mölstad et al. 2002), the aim of this study is to shed light on potential underlying linguistic and culture-bound causes for this difference, and the interplay between the linguistic and cultural dimensions. This study takes a comprehensive approach, examining the actions and attitudes of the three groups of 'stakeholders' in the way antibiotics are prescribed: prescriber, patient, and health policy decision-makers.

According to the World Health Organization (WHO), antibiotic resistance has become a major health issue. In 2015, a global action plan was endorsed in order to tackle the problems of antibiotic resistance and to ensure continuity of successful medical treatment (*Global action plan on antimicrobial resistance* 2015). As a supplement to the global initiative,

K. A. J. Kragh (✉) • E. Strudsholm
Department of English, Germanic and Romance Studies, University of Copenhagen, Copenhagen, Denmark
e-mail: kirstenkragh@hum.ku.dk; struds@hum.ku.dk

C. S. Jensen et al. (eds.), *Risking Antimicrobial Resistance*,
https://doi.org/10.1007/978-3-319-90656-0_3

the EU, acting within the framework of European Centre for Disease Preventions and Control (ECDC), has since 2008 launched the annual European Antibiotic Awareness Day in order to 'raise awareness about the threat to public health of antibiotic resistance and the importance of prudent antibiotic use' (*European Antibiotic Awareness Day* 2005–2017).

Our study describes the current state of affairs in France and Italy and compares this to Denmark in terms of governmental initiatives and regulations regarding antibiotic resistance. We examine how the European health initiative European Antibiotic Awareness Day is carried out in France and Italy as compared to Denmark and the relative impact of this initiative in pursuing antibiotic resistance in the three countries. In analysing the medical practice in the three countries, we take a linguistic perspective. We focus on the information given to doctors and patients, respectively, in order to assess how different national approaches influence prescribers' and patients' inclination to choose antibiotic treatment. Our hypothesis is that the linguistic and cultural features of each country affect the prescription behaviour, and conversely, that differences in behaviour reflect cultural and linguistic differences.

3.2 Antimicrobial Resistance in Global, European, and National Perspectives

As early as 1960, Japanese scientists were aware that bacteria which had become resistant could transfer the resistibility to other bacteria, including the transmission of resistance from animals to humans. However, it would take another decade or more before the awareness of this health-threatening development became a public issue. Until then, veterinarian authorities were under continuous pressure to liberalize the prescription of antibiotics to promote 'efficient farming' (Bavnhøj 1977). In Denmark, the earliest signs of public awareness appeared when the Danish environmental movement, in 1978, published a poster of a pig with the words: 'Danish pigs are healthy and full of penicillin'. With Denmark being a major producer and exporter of pork products, the Danish co-operative slaughterhouses tried to halt the campaign in court. The graphic designer,

Michael Witte, who was the instigator of the poster, created a series of posters on the same theme along with the progress of the trial, which ended with a 1980 Supreme Court decision acquitting Witte. In addition to calling attention to the use of penicillin within Denmark, the campaign had international echoes (*DEN-1980-X-002* 1980).

According to a study from 2001 (Cars et al. 2001), *sales* of antibiotics vary significantly from country to country, expressed in daily doses per 1000 people. France seems to have the highest use, reaching 36.51 doses per 1000; this is compared with Italy's 23.99 and Denmark's 11.35. A parallel source presenting data based on antibiotic *prescriptions* per 1000 inhabitants show that France, in 1997, had 1041 per thousand compared to 964 in Italy and only 525 in Denmark. More recent studies containing data from 2015 show the same tendency: 16.1 daily doses per 1000 inhabitants in Denmark, 29.9 in France, and 27.5 in Italy (*Summary of the latest data on antibiotic consumption in the European Union* 2016). When we look at the resistance rate, the overall tendency is that Italy is by far the country with the greatest resistance problems (25 to 50 per cent of occurrences of a given bacterium not responding to antibiotic treatment), Denmark is the country with the lowest resistance percentage (one to five per cent), while France (around 10 to 15 per cent on average) is in between, closer to Denmark than to Italy (*Summary of the latest data on antibiotic resistance in the European Union* 2016).

Medical studies indicate a clear relationship between the level of awareness of appropriate use of antibiotics and the level of resistance (Earnshaw et al. 2009). It is therefore remarkable that France has such a high level of antibiotic consumption, even higher than Italy, but has nevertheless a much lower rate of resistance. The great difference between the countries has led to radical initiatives at all levels, from worldwide to national and regional programs.

WHO is involved in implementing a global strategy and guidelines for countries that want to monitor resistance to antibiotics and take effective action. As part of this strategy, the first World Antibiotic Awareness Week was held from 16 to 22 November 2015. The campaign aims to increase awareness of global antibiotic resistance and to encourage best practices among the general public, health workers, and policy-makers in order to avoid the growth and spread of antibiotic resistance. Prior to this campaign, the WHO, in May 2015, published a *Global Action Plan on Antimicrobial Resistance*, which aimed at improving awareness regarding both human and animal consumption, enhancing research and its dissemination, reducing the incidence of infections through increased focus on sanitation and hygiene, and involving all countries regardless of economic conditions. Furthermore, one result of the awareness day was a manual for developing national action plans to address antimicrobial resistance. This manual 'proposes an incremental approach that countries can adapt to the specific needs, circumstances and available resources of each individual country' (*Antimicrobial resistance. A manual for developing national action plans* 2016).

Although legislation on health matters is not governed by the European Union (EU), The Council of the European Union, in 2001, published a set of recommendations on the prudent use of antimicrobial agents in human medicine based on a resolution from 1999 concerning a strategy against the microbial threat (*Council Recommendation of 15 November 2001 on the prudent use of antimicrobial agents in human medicine* 2001). This is underscored by the European Antibiotic Awareness Day, which is facilitated and disseminated by the EU and which since 2008 has taken place either as a day or as a full week dedicated to the awareness of the threat of antibiotic resistance. The homepage for the European Antibiotic Awareness Day offers information in all the official EU languages. Thus, we find the same information in the same pamphlets with the same graphic design and similar rhetoric in French, Italian, and Danish. When the same effort is made to create awareness of the correct use of antibiotics, the question can be raised: Why is antibiotic resistance a problem of different proportions in the three countries?

3.3 The Scope of Linguistic and Cultural Dimensions

The theoretical framework of our approach is based on the interplay between cultural and linguistic dimensions, and our intention is to shed light on the relation between differences in behaviour and linguistic and cultural differences. These perspectives take their point of departure on insights into cognitive interdependence of language and culture, and on the interaction between innate/universal and culture-bound/particular linguistic competencies that arise from these. We hypothesize that the high level of antibiotic resistance in Southern Europe compared to the North is related to differences in information culture and more specifically, to the differing types of relations between the prescriber and user (doctor–patient) in the three countries.

Deschepper et al. (2008) have discussed whether 'culture dimensions [are] relevant for explaining cross-national differences in antibiotic use in Europe'. Taking their point of departure in Hofstede's model of cultural dimensions, they conclude that 'the culture-specific way in which people deal with authority is an important factor in explaining cross-national differences in antibiotic use'. In Hofstede's model, countries are classified according to a list of cultural dimensions, including *power distance*, *uncertainty avoidance*, *individualism versus collectivism*, and *masculinity versus femininity*, of which power distance is particularly relevant for our approach. Power distance concerns the unequal distribution of power in a society and the extent to which the population accepts this hierarchical order. In high-power-distance countries, doctors are highly respected by patients, while in low-power-distance countries, doctors and patients tend to consider each other as roughly social equals. In the interpretation of Hofstede's model suggested by Verma et al. (2016), the Nordic countries belong to the low-power-distance societies, while Latin countries (France and Italy) are generally high-power-distance communities. Furthermore, we refer to Perkins (1992), who analyses the relation between culture-bound and linguistic properties by considering a dialogue as a culture-bound situation (see also Kragh and Strudsholm 2015).

Taking our point of departure in this theoretical framework, and with reference to our hypothesis according to which both linguistic and cultural features of each nationality affect the behaviour, and that different behaviours reflect cultural and linguistic differences, we propose to analyse the existing guidelines to prescribers and consumers and to see how the effect of these guidelines reflects linguistic and cultural differences.

After an overview of the development of consumption and antimicrobial resistance in the three countries, we take a linguistic and comparative approach to a selection of information material from the ECDC. On the surface, the information materials are identical, but closer examination reveals subtle linguistic differences that may reflect culture-based factors. This raises the question of whether it makes sense to use the same information materials and guidelines in countries and cultures with different levels of the resistance problem. Although the communication situations are basically the same, they will appear differently in the three languages because they represent different cultural and mental universes. This will be further developed in Sect. 3.4.4.

3.4 Analysis

The European initiatives have given rise to national programs and campaigns aimed at enhancing awareness of the increasing resistance. Out of EU's 28 member states, only 13 have an action plan for antibiotic resistance. Among these are Denmark (*Fælles antibiotika- og resistenshandlingsplan* 2010) and France (*Plan national d'alerte sur les antibiotiques 2011–2016* 2011), while Italy has no national action plan (*Antimicrobial resistance strategies and action plans* 2016). Health regulations in Italy are to a large extent delegated to regional governments. In the following, we will look into local conditions of antimicrobial resistance policy in the three countries.

3.4.1 Denmark

Until recently, Denmark was the European country with the lowest antibiotic consumption. This is no longer the case. Consumption has increased in Denmark and decreased in certain other countries. Nonetheless, Danish antibiotic consumption remains much lower than in many other countries. 90 per cent of the antibiotics used are prescribed by the primary sector, that is by general practitioners. Since 2011, it appears that the level of consumption has stabilized, and in the primary sector, the number of prescriptions and of treated patients has even dropped.

The consumption is kept under surveillance by Statens Serum Institut (The Danish National Serum Institute), which provides data for the

European Antimicrobial Resistance Surveillance Network (EARS-Net) and the European Surveillance of Antimicrobial Consumption Network (ESAC-Net).

3.4.2 France

In 2000, France was the European country with the highest antibiotic consumption, with 36 daily intakes per 1000 inhabitants, considerably higher than the European average of 21 daily doses per 1000 inhabitants (Rasi et al. 2009; Pepin and Ricordeau 2006). Since then, France has made great progress, and the years 2002–2007 saw consumption reduced by 23.4 per cent.

In France, three major plans have been carried out, starting with the *Plan d'action pluriannuel* 2001–2005. This plan was extended and completed by the *Plan 2007–2010* (*Plan antibiotiques 2007–2010: propositions du Comité de suivi pour la deuxième phase du Plan pour préserver l'efficacité des antibiotiques* 2007), which the earlier plan sought to control and rationalize the prescription of antibiotics in order to maintain their effectiveness. In continuation of these two national plans, a third strategy (*Plan national d'alerte sur les antibiotiques 2011–2016* 2011) was launched, the aim of which was to counter the increasing resistance to antibiotics. This third campaign focuses more on how to prevent situations where prescribers feel obliged to prescribe antibiotics, including situations where there is no evidence of susceptible bacteria. This campaign seeks to engage all groups involved in the cycle of antibiotic consumption: patients, their families, healthcare professionals of all levels, researchers, institutions, and so on. The objective is to reduce antibiotic consumption by 25 per cent in five years. The plan comprises three major goals: improving relations between doctor and patient, preserving the effectiveness of antibiotics, and promoting further research in the field.

3.4.3 Italy

The analyses published in *Rapporto sull'uso dei farmaci antibiotici* (Rasi et al. 2009) show a 13 per cent growth in consumption of antibiotics in

Italy during the period 1999–2007. Compared to other European countries, Italy has Europe's third highest consumption of antibiotics, after France and Cyprus, and twice the consumption of Germany and the UK.

A national campaign from 2010, entitled *Antibiotici. Difendi la tua difesa. Usali con cautela* (Antibiotics. Defend your defense. Use them with caution) is aimed at informing citizens about the importance of resorting to antibiotics only when necessary and when they are prescribed by a doctor. However, consumption of antibiotics at regional levels shows a wide variability in Italy, with increasing gradients of consumption from North to South. The lowest consumption rates are in Northern Italy compared to double the average consumption in Southern Italy.

3.4.4 Analysis of Selected Informative Material

According to EU default language policy, informative material is produced in all EU languages at the same time, following the EU's principle of 'respect[ing] its rich cultural and linguistic diversity' (*Fact Sheets on the European Union: Language policy* 2017). In principle, no EU language is superior to another. However, since detailed information is often published only in English and French, these two languages may possibly act as source languages for translation into the other languages. As there is no official statement on these matters, and since there is no trace in the analysed material that indicates direct translation of English/French into Danish or Italian, this possibility will not be taken further into account. One can thus expect the texts to be parallel.

The homepages of the European Antibiotic Awareness Day in the three different languages indicate different ways of approaching the consumer (*European Antibiotic Awareness Day* 2005–2017 and parallel pages in Danish, French, and Italian). This material has been prepared centrally by the EU initiative and appears in all European languages. In the following, English is included as a *TERTIUM COMPARATIONIS* (base comparison) and in order to avoid repetitive translations. The diversity of the titles in the different languages indicates that neither English nor French is the source language. As shown in Table 3.1, the English text mentions the word

Table 3.1 Forms used in the material from the European Antibiotic Awareness Day

English	Danish	French	Italian
European Antibiotic Awareness Day	Europæisk Antibiotikadag	Journée Européenne d'information sur les antibiotiques	Giornata europea degli antibiotici
Plan a campaign	Planlægning af en kampagne	Préparer une campagne	Progettare una campagne
Get informed	Få information	S'informer	Cosa dovete sapere
Get involved	Vær med!	Participer	Partecipate alla campagna

'awareness' while the French focuses on 'information'. Neither of these two words is reproduced in the Danish and the Italian versions shown in Table 3.1.

The material consists mostly of guidelines for prescribers and patients expressed in different linguistic forms, among these obviously the imperative mood. The Danish verbal system has only one imperative form which is used for both singular and plural and informal and formal contexts. French has two imperative forms, second person singular and second person plural. The singular is used among friends and family addressed to a single person, and the plural form likewise is used to address two or more persons. Furthermore, the plural form is used in approaches to one or more persons in less informal situations. In addition, French uses the infinitive form as an alternative to the imperative in more formal contexts to indicate an impersonal command to an unknown audience, especially in warnings and instruction manuals, but also in less formal genres such as recipes. Like the French system, the Italian verbal system has imperative forms in the second person singular and plural, but they are both informal, with no distinction for formality, only of number. In addition, Italian has imperatives in the third person singular and plural, identical with the subjunctive forms, which are used in formal communication. Moreover, Italian uses the infinitive form in the same way as French (Skytte 1983; Weinrich 1982).

The Danish version of *Plan a campaign* is a nominal construction *Planlægning af en kampagne* 'planning of a campaign', a form which does not have the same sense of involvement as the French and Italian infinitives *Préparer*/*Progettare*. In the Danish versions of *Get informed* and *Get involved*, the consumer is addressed by the imperatives *Få information* and *Vær med!* In the French version, the consumer is addressed by the infinitives *S'informer* 'inform oneself' and *Participer* 'participate'. The Italian version presents an interrogative construction *Cosa dovete sapere*, literally 'what do you ought to know' and an imperative *Participate alla campagna* 'Take part in the campaign' which is parallel to the Danish version. The use of the imperative in Danish and Italian and of the present indicative second person plural in Italian is more personal and signals informality, while the use of the infinitive in French signals impersonality and formality. However, the Italian phrasing *Cosa dovete sapere*, with the modal verb *dovere* 'ought to', contains an element of morality. It is more regulative and educating than the Danish and French versions.

Our observations point towards a difference in the level of formality in which Danish and Italian constitute an informal structure, and French a more formal character. This is remarkable, since one could have expected the two Romance languages to act similarly in contrast to Danish. In the following, we will take a linguistic look at the material found in the underlying websites. We will focus on the guidelines for primary care prescribers on how to communicate with the patient and on a leaflet that primary care prescribers should distribute to patients. Our purpose is to examine whether this tendency of differences in formality can be further confirmed.

3.4.4.1 Information to Prescribers

According to the ECDC, communication with the patients is of great importance, and professional consultancy containing realistic expectations about the progress of the disease has a greater impact on the patient's satisfaction than prescription of antibiotics (European Antibiotic Awareness Day 2005–2017).

Prescribers are offered 'A model for a patient dialogue on the basis of available evidence' which 'provides guidance and support for primary care prescribers who encounter patient pressure for antibiotics, and promotes appropriate antibiotic use by patients' (*Material for primary care prescribers* 2005–2017). On the surface, this model seems to be entirely the same in the three languages analysed here, but when looking more closely at some linguistic features, differences appear, as shown in Table 3.2 (the words in bold have been emphasized by the authors).

In the patient's parts of the dialogue, we cannot identify any significant differences. In all three languages, the phrases are in the third person singular, present tense, referring to the patient (*Relaterer/Précise/Racconta*, *Beskriver/Décrit/Descrive*, *Kræver/Demande/Chiede*, *Spørger/S'informe/Ch iede*).

In the doctor's part of the dialogue, however, we find both intralinguistic and interlinguistic differences, especially as regards type of modality expressed in the verbal forms. In Danish, the imperative form is used consistently in the graphic presentation of the doctor–patient dialogue: *Spørg*, *Ordiner*, *Informer*, *Bekræft*. In contrast, in the corresponding contexts, French and Italian use the infinitive forms (*Demander/Chiedere*, *Préscrire/Prescrivere*, *Fornire*, *Confermare*). It is remarkable that the French version, after this use of the infinitive form, uses the second person singular of the imperative (*Donne*, *Confirme*) and not the infinitive form, nor the second person plural form of the imperative. The change from infinitive to second person singular imperative takes place from the point of deciding whether or not to prescribe. Thus, we observe a movement from formal to less formal in the approach to the prescriber. In the Italian version, the infinitive form is used in all four examples.

In the third box, which again speaks to the doctor, the choice of verbal form has been avoided in the Danish and Italian versions by nominalization (*Drøftelse*, *Discussione*), while the French version maintains the infinitive (*Discuter*). This could indicate a deontic modality in the French version, whereas the nominalizations in Danish and Italian are more neutral.

In the last part of the dialogue, the prescriber is advised to *confirm that the patient has understood and agrees with management strategy*. The use of the infinitive (*confermare*) and the subjunctive (*abbia*) in the Italian model suggests a more distant and formal communication between doctor and patient than in the Danish and French models.

Table 3.2 Examples from the guidelines for patient—prescriber dialogue

Agent	English	Danish	French	Italian
Doctor	Enquires about patient symptoms	**Spørg** til patientens symptomer	**Demander** au patient quels sont ses symptômes	**Chiedere** i sintomi al paziente
Patient	Relates history of present illness/ describes past medical history and risk factors	**Relaterer** til tidligere sygdom i anamnesen/**Beskriver** tidligere anamnese og risikofaktorer	**Précise** l'histoire de la maladie actuelle/**Décrit** les antécédents médicaux et les facteurs de risques	**Racconta** la storia della malattia attuale/ **Descrive** l'anamnesi e i fattori di rischio
Doctor	Discussion of patient illness and options for management plan	**Drøftelse** af patientsygdom og muligheder for behandlingsplan	**Discuter** de la maladie du patient et des options de prise en charge	**Discussione** sulla malattia del paziente e sulle opzioni terapeutiche
Doctor	DO NOT PRESCRIBE ANTIBIOTICS	**ORDINER** IKKE ANTIBIOTIKA	NE PAS **PRESCRIRE** DES ANTIBIOTIQUES	NON **PRESCRIVERE** ANTIBIOTICI
Doctor	PRESCRIBE ANTIBIOTICS	**ORDINER** ANTIBIOTIKA	**PRESCRIRE** DES ANTIBIOTIQUES	**PRESCRIVERE** ANTIBIOTICI
Patient	Demands antibiotics/ Enquires about non-antibiotic treatments	**Kræver** antibiotika/**Spørger** til andre behandlinger end antibiotikabehandlinger	**Demande** des antibiotiques/**S'informe** sur les traitements non antibiotiques	**Chiede** antibiotici/**Chiede** informazioni sulle terapie non basate su antibiotici
Doctor	Provides information about antibiotic resistance, potential benefits and side-effects of antibiotics	**Informer** om antibiotikaresistens, potentielle fordele og bivirkninger ved antibiotika	**Donne** des informations sur la résistance aux antibiotiques, les bénéfices potentiels let les effets secondaires des antibiotiques	**Fornire** informazioni sulla resistenza agli antiotici, sui possibili benefici ed effetti collaterali degli antibiotici
Doctor	Confirms that patient has understood and agrees with management strategy	**Bekræft**, at patienten har forstået og er enig i behandlingsstrategien	**Confirme** que le patient a compris et qu'il accepte la stratégie de prise en charge	**Confermare** che il paziente abbia compreso e accettato la strategia terapeutica

On one hand, we find common tendencies of French and Italian in opposition to Danish in line with the traditional linguistic classification. On the other hand, we observe a new opposition of Danish and French against Italian. These observations suggest that such variations are not entirely linguistic.

3.4.4.2 Information to Patients/Consumers

A closer look at the underlying *Factsheet for general public* (2005–2017), containing information aimed at patients, reveals the same type of marginal linguistic differences, see Table 3.3.

The deontic aspect of appeal in the Danish version is expressed by a direct approach to consumers by using the imperative form and the pronouns in the second person singular (*du, dine*). The French and Italian versions use the impersonal infinitive construction. Thus, the approach to Danish consumers is very direct (*Vask dine og dine børns hænder*), whereas the approach to French and Italian consumers is impersonal and less including. This difference between Danish and the two Romance languages reflects the common understanding of different levels of formality and reflects cultural differences (Kragh et al. 2016). This diversity continues in the underlying pages (*Get informed* 2005–2017), see Table 3.4.

Here the Danish and the Italian versions share common informal features, with the imperative form in the last sentence (Da. *Se*, It. *Leggete*). In contrast, the French version is more formal, with the impersonal interrogative construction with the infinitive (*Comment utiliser*) and the omission of the verb in the last sequence (*Témoignages de patients*). Common to the French and Italian versions is the use of the word *responsable*/*responsabile* in a sentence which is left out of the Danish version. This word appeals to the patients' responsibility, in opposition to the prior sentence, where the words *prudente*, *prudente*, and *fornuftig* invoke common sense. Apparently, it was not deemed necessary to explicate the meaning of prudent use to Danes. Could the Southern European appeal to responsibility versus the Northern common-sense approach indicate a contrast between individuality and community?

Table 3.3 Examples from Factsheets for general public

English	Danish	French	Italian
Follow your doctor's advice when taking antibiotics	**Følg** lægens råd, når **du** tager antibiotika	**Suivre** les recommandations du médecin qui leur a prescrit des antibiotiques	**Seguire** le indicazioni del medico sull'assunzione degli antibiotici
When possible, prevent infection through appropriate vaccination	**Sørg** for, når det er muligt, at forhindre infektion via relevant vaccination	Si possible, **éviter** les infections en procédant à des vaccinations appropriées	Se possibile, **prevenire** le infezioni attraverso le vaccinazioni
Wash your hands and your children's hands regularly, for instance after sneezing or coughing before touching other things or people	**Vask dine** og **dine** børns hænder regelmæssigt, for eksempel efter nys eller host, før **du** rører ved andre ting eller mennesker	Se **laver** les mains et laver les mains des enfants régulièrement, notamment suite à un éternuement ou une quinte de toux, avant de toucher des objets ou d'autres personnes	**Lavarsi** sempre le mani e assicurarsi che anche i bambini lo facciano, ad esempio dopo aver starnutito o tossito e prima di toccare cose o persone
Always use antibiotics under medical prescription, not using 'leftovers' or antibiotics obtained without a prescription	**Brug** altid antibiotika på recept og undgå at bruge 'rester' eller antibiotika uden recept	Toujours se **conformer** à la prescription médicale lors de la prise d'antibiotiques. Ne pas utiliser les «restes» de l'armoire à pharmacie ou bien des antibiotiques obtenus sans ordonnance	**Usare** solo gli antibiotici specificamente prescritti dal medico e non gli antibiotici rimasti da una terapia precedente oppure ottenuti senza ricetta
Ask your pharmacist about how to dispose of the remaining medicines	**Spørg** på apoteket, hvad **du** skal gøre ved medicinrester	**Demander** au pharmacien comment jeter les médicaments inutilisés	**Chiedere** al farmacista come smaltire i medicinali non utilizzati

Table 3.4 Examples from the underlying pages 'Get informed'

English	Danish	French	Italian
What is antibiotic resistance and prudent antibiotic use? How to use antibiotics responsibly? See patient stories, infographics, videos	Hvad er antibiotikaresistens og **fornuftig** brug af antibiotika? **Se** patienthistorier, infografik og videoer	Qu'est-ce que la résistance aux antibiotiques et l'utilisation **prudente** des antibiotiques ? **Comment utiliser** les antibiotiques de façon **responsable** ? **Témoignages de patients**, infographies et vidéos	Che cos'è la resistenza agli antibiotici e cosa si intende con "uso **prudente**" degli antibiotici? Come si usano gli antibiotici in maniera **responsabile**? **Leggete** le storie dei pazienti, guardate le infografiche e i video

In the following, we will discuss whether these linguistic differences could indicate some culture-bound differences that may help explain why Italy, in spite of the more limited consumption than France, has more antibiotic resistance than France, and why France in turn, has more serious problems with antibiotic resistance than Denmark.

3.5 Discussion: Cultural Dimensions

The European Antibiotic Awareness Day presents guidelines for the dialogue between doctor and patient in exactly the same diagrammatic form for all involved nations, that is all EU languages; however, we have noticed slight linguistic differences with regard to the code related to the given culture. Among Hofstede's parameters of cultural dimensions, we find three dimensions to be especially pertinent, namely power distance (use of antibiotics), masculinity, and uncertainty avoidance (that the doctor prescribes antibiotics to avoid uncertainty about the diagnosis). These differences are shown in Table 3.5.

These three parameters correlate partially and mutually reinforce each other. The power distance score is relatively high in France and Italy,

Table 3.5 Dimensions expressed on a scale from 0 to 100

Dimension type (after Hoftstede)	Denmark	France	Italy
Power distance	18	68	50
Masculinity	16	43	70
Uncertainty avoidance	23	86	75

indicating a hierarchical relation between doctor and patient and consequently a more formal dialogue, while the lower score in Denmark corresponds well with the Danish societal structure of equality. Thus, Denmark's position in the low rank of the power distance dimension reflects characteristic features of Danish society, such as employee autonomy, informal atmosphere, direct and involving communication, and also between doctor and patient (*Geert Hofstede* 2017). In France, by contrast, relations between parents and children, doctors and patients, as well as between employers and employees, are characterized by dependency and acceptance of inequality. In Italy, there is a clear distinction between North and South: the society of Northern Italy resembles Northern European countries, with equality and decentralization of power and decision-making, whereas the higher score in Southern Italy reflects the opposite. A different way of interpreting the impact of power distance is suggested by Murray et al. (2011), who discuss the different values of obedience in the different cultures, and take obedience as an indication of power distance. The scores of masculinity correlate in general with power distance, but it should be noted that the masculinity factor points in both directions. In countries where both men and women are working outside the home, there is a tendency for people not to allow themselves or their children to be absent from work or school, which could lead to more antibiotic prescriptions. On the other hand, feminine cultures such as Denmark are more concerned with ecological problems, which again triggers more prudent consumption to prevent resistance (Deschepper et al. 2008). The medium score of France reflects a unique culture not found elsewhere, with a feminine upper class and a masculine working class. The high score on masculinity in Italy corresponds well to the competitive and success-oriented society. Frellick (2015) cites Dr. Michael Borg from Malta, a country with a high level of antibiotic resistance, according to whom 'It's not the prescribing we have to address, it's the behaviour'. Borg, whose research is inspired by two of Hofstede's factors, power distance and uncertainty avoidance, defines responsible use of antibiotics as 'choosing the correct antibiotic for the appropriate indication in the correct dose at the right time'. In this context, it is interesting that both the French and the Italian sites use the word *responsible/responsabile*. In countries with a high score on the third parameter, uncertainty avoidance, doctors tend to prescribe more antibiotics to reduce the feeling of uncertainty of diagnosis. Cultures with high power distance and masculinity do not expect uncertainty from the doctor. Studies by Watkins et al. (2015), for instance, indicate that Hispanics in the USA have a higher consumption of antibiotics than average, which corresponds well with the idea of cultural norms related to the Spanish-speaking world. This suggests that even outside the national frames, the original culture and language influence the consumption pattern. Watkins et al. (2015) advocate the use of 'culturally appropriate materials in both English and Spanish', underscoring the continuous need of information material adapted to specific cultures.

3.6 Conclusions and Perspectives

We have analysed information material from three countries with different levels of antibiotic resistance. In spite of increasing antibiotic consumption in Denmark, the level of antimicrobial resistance remains low. France has a higher level of consumption than Italy, but a lower level of resistance. According to our hypothesis, these differences can be culture-bound, and our aim has been to examine whether the existing information materials in the three languages reflect such differences in their linguistic codes. In addition to the obvious language-specific differences (French and Italian versus Danish), we have found differences in the morpho-syntactic structure, by which the use of different verb forms (imperatives, infinitives, and verbal nouns) correlates with different levels of formality. These distinctions reflect some of the culture-bound dimensions presented by Hofstede and support the hypothesis of a correlation between the level of antibiotic resistance and culture-bound linguistic variation. These differences could have been much better reflected in the studied material which has proven to be far too uniform, with no consideration of cultural dimensions in linguistic behaviour (Kragh et al. 2016). Differences in power distance and uncertainty avoidance are not considered, and these differences may help explain the differences among the three countries.

References

Bavnhøj, H. J. (1977). Om dyrlægers placering i forbrugersamfundets produktions-, effektivitets- og profitræs. *Dansk Veterinærtidsskrift, 60,* 124–127.

Cars, O., Mölstad, S., & Melander, A. (2001). Variation in antibiotic use in the European Union. *The Lancet, 357,* 1851–1853.

Deschepper, R., Grigoryan, L., Lundborg, C. S., Hofstede, G., Cohen, J., Van Der Kelen, G., … Haaijer-Ruskamp, F. M. (2008). Are cultural dimensions relevant for explaining cross-national differences in antibiotic use in Europe? *BMC Health Services Research, 8,* 123.

Earnshaw, S., Monnet, D. L., Duncan, B., O'Toole, J., Ekdahl, K., & Goossens, H. (2009). European Antibiotic Awareness Day, 2008—The first Europe-wide public information campaign on prudent antibiotic use: Methods and survey of activities in participating countries. *Eurosurveillance, 14*(30), 19280.

Frellick, M. (2015). Antibiotic resistance powered by cultural norms. *Medscape.* https://www.medscape.com/viewarticle/843859

Kragh, K. J., Skafte Jensen, E., & Strudsholm, E. (2016). Åbninger og lukninger i e-mailkorrespondance på fire sprog. *Globe: A Journal of Language, Culture and Communication, Special issue 1,* 119–139.

Kragh, K. J., & Strudsholm, E. (2015). Deiksis i sprog og kontekst. Deiktiske relativsætninger i et komparativt, kognitivt perspektiv. *Skandinaviske sprogstudier, 6,* 134–157.

Mölstad, S., Lundborg, C. S., Karlsson, A.-K., & Cars, O. (2002). Antibiotic prescription rates vary markedly between 13 European countries. *Infectious Diseases, 34,* 366–371.

Murray, D. R., Trudeau, R., & Schaller, M. (2011). On the origins of cultural differences in conformity: Four tests of the pathogen prevalence hypothesis. *Personality and Social Psychology Bulletin, 37,* 318–329.

Pepin, S., & Ricordeau, P. (2006). La consommation d'antibiotiques: Situation en France au regard des autres pays européens. *Points de repère, 6,* 1–8.

Perkins, R. D. (1992). *Deixis, grammar, and culture.* Amsterdam/Philadelphia: John Benjamins Publishing Company.

Rasi, G., Gallo, P. F., Gasparini, A., Masiero, L., & Montilla, S. (2009). *Rapporto sull'uso dei farmaci antibiotici. Analisi del consumo territoriale nelle regioni italiane*. Roma: Agenzia Italiana del Farmaco.

Skytte, G. (1983). *La sintassi dell'infinito in italiano moderno*. København: Munksgaards Forlag.

Verma, A., Griffin, A., Dacre, J., & Elder, A. (2016). Exploring cultural and linguistic influences on clinical communication skills: A qualitative study of International Medical Graduates. *BMC Medical Education, 16*, 162.

Watkins, L. K. F., Sanchez, G. V., Albert, A. P., Roberts, R. M., & Hicks, L. A. (2015). Knowledge and attitudes regarding antibiotic use among adult consumers, adult hispanic consumers, and health care providers—United States, 2012–2013. *Weekly, 64*, 767–770.

Weinrich, H. (1982). *Textgrammatik der französischen Sprache*. Stuttgart: Ernst Klett Verlag.

Consulted Webpages

Antibiotici. Difendi la tua difesa. Usali con cautela [Online]. 2010. Agenzia Italiana del Farmaco. Retrieved April 2017, from http://www.agenziafarmaco.gov.it/it/content/antibiotici-difendi-la-tua-difesa-usali-con-cautela-0

Antimicrobial resistance strategies and action plans [Online]. 2016. European Centre for Disease Prevention and Control. Retrieved April 2017, from http://ecdc.europa.eu/en/healthtopics/Healthcare-associated_infections/guidance-infection-prevention-control/Pages/antimicrobial-resistance-strategies-action-plans.aspx

Antimicrobial resistance. A manual for developing national action plans [Online]. 2016. World Health Organization. Retrieved April 2017, from http://www.who.int/drugresistance/action-plans/manual/en/

Council Recommendation of 15 November 2001 on the prudent use of antimicrobial agents in human medicine [Online]. 2001. Brussels: European Commission. Retrieved April 2017, from http://eur-lex.europa.eu/legal-content/EN/TXT/PDF/?uri=CELEX:32002H0077&rid=2.

DEN-1980-X-002 [Online]. 1980. Retrieved April 2017, from http://www.codices.coe.int/NXT/gateway.dll/CODICES/full/eur/den/den/den-1980-x-002?fn=document-frame.htm$f=templates$3.0

European Antibiotic Awareness Day [Online]. 2005–2017. European Centre for Disease Prevention and Control. Retrieved April 2017, from http://ecdc.europa.eu/en/EAAD/Pages/Home.aspx/.

Fact Sheets on the European Union: Language policy [Online]. 2017. European Parliament. Retrieved April 2017, from http://www.europarl.europa.eu/atyourservice/en/displayFtu.html?ftuId=FTU_5.13.6.html

Factsheet for general public [Online]. 2005–2017. European Centre for Disease Prevention and Control. Retrieved April 2017, from http://ecdc.europa.eu/en/eaad/antibiotics-get-informed/factsheets/Pages/general-public.aspx

Fælles antibiotika- og resistenshandlingsplan [Online]. 2010. Indenrigs- og Sundhedsministeriet. Ministeriet for Fødevarer, Landbrug og Fiskeri. Retrieved March 2017, from http://www.sum.dk/Aktuelt/Nyheder/Sundhedspolitik/2010/Maj/~/media/Filer-dokumenter/Antibiotikaresistens/Handlingsplan_mod_antibiotikaresistens.ashx

Geert Hofstede [Online]. 2017. Retrieved April 2017, from https://geert-hofstede.com/denmark.html

Get informed [Online]. 2005–2017. European Centre for Disease Prevention and Control. Retrieved April 2017, from http://ecdc.europa.eu/en/eaad/antibiotics-get-informed/Pages/get-informed.aspx

Global action plan on antimicrobial resistance [Online]. 2015. World Heath Organization. Retrieved January 2017, from http://www.who.int/antimicrobial-resistance/publications/global-action-plan/en/

Material for primary care prescribers [Online]. 2005–2017. European Centre for Disease Prevention and Control. Retrieved April 2017, from http://ecdc.europa.eu/en/eaad/antibiotics-info-prescribers/material-primary-care-prescribers/Pages/material-primary-care-prescribers.aspx

Plan antibiotiques 2007–2010: Propositions du Comité de suivi pour la deuxième phase du Plan pour préserver l'efficacité des antibiotiques [Online]. 2007. Retrieved April 2017, from http://www.plan-antibiotiques.sante.gouv.fr/IMG/pdf/bilan_plan_2007.pdf

Plan national d'alerte sur les antibiotiques 2011–2016 [Online]. 2011. Ministère du travail, de l'emploi et de la santé. Retrieved April 2017, from http://social-sante.gouv.fr/IMG/pdf/plan_antibiotiques_2011–2016_DEFINITIF.pdf

Summary of the latest data on antibiotic consumption in the European Union [Online]. 2016. Stockholm: European Centre for Disease Prevention and Control. Retrieved April 2017, from http://ecdc.europa.eu/en/eaad/Documents/antibiotics-consumption-EU-data-2014.pdf

Summary of the latest data on antibiotic resistance in the European Union [Online]. 2016. Stockholm: European Centre for Disease Prevention and Control. Retrieved April 2017, from http://ecdc.europa.eu/en/eaad/Documents/antibiotics-consumption-EU-data-2014.pdf

4

Talk on Cough: Symptom, Sign and Significance in Acute Primary Care

Johanna Lindell

4.1 Introduction: Addressing the Symptom of Cough

Acute bronchitis, a cough persisting for several days to weeks, has been found to be one of the most common reasons for prescribing antibiotics for lower respiratory tract infections, especially in primary care (Cals et al. 2009). However, as the infections are predominantly viral, most of these prescriptions do not benefit the patient (Wigton et al. 2008). Treating viral infections with antibiotics is unnecessary, costly, and a health risk in the short and long term, especially because of the risk of resistance.

While cough and especially its overtreatment have been studied, authentic communication on cough has not been closely studied as an interactional phenomenon on its own. Analysing data from the particular Danish context, where the overall prescribing rates remain low, this chapter investigates how Danish general practitioners (GPs) and patients

J. Lindell (✉)
Department of Nordic Studies and Linguistics, University of Copenhagen, Copenhagen, Denmark
e-mail: dbm661@hum.ku.dk

C. S. Jensen et al. (eds.), *Risking Antimicrobial Resistance*,
https://doi.org/10.1007/978-3-319-90656-0_4

reach agreement on non-antibiotic treatment when patients present with cough. It focuses specifically on symptom residue sequences—symptoms left unexplained by the diagnosis (Frankel 2001; Maynard and Frankel 2006; see also Beach et al. 2005). Introducing and re-introducing a symptom such as cough after a diagnosis or treatment recommendation suggests that to this patient, the symptom may pose a health risk. Several scholars have shown that responding more than minimally to diagnosis and responses other than acceptance of a treatment recommendation are treated by physicians as resistance even when there may be a request for more information, reassurance, or specific actions (Heath 1992; Peräkylä 1998, 2002; Stivers 2007). In cases of respiratory tract infections, such resistance has been shown to increase physician perception of pressure for antibiotics (Mangione-Smith et al. 2006). In addition, if GPs do not address the patient′s perception of the symptom and the risk it poses, patients may seek medical aid again for similar symptoms. Both could lead to unnecessary prescribing. This chapter investigates how the orientation to cough, as a subjective symptom of illness or a sign of disease, can influence prescription decisions and how such pressure may be navigated without leading to unnecessary use of antibiotics.

In the following sections, I will first introduce the different understandings of symptoms as they are raised in the consultation. Building on the specific data available for this chapter, I will then analyse how and when cough and its accompanying symptoms are re-introduced by patients and how GPs respond to this. I will then discuss the import of these findings on antibiotic prescribing practices.

4.2 Negotiating the Significance of a Symptom

The discrepancy and overlaps between physicians' primary concern for disease (biomedical diagnosis) and patients' primary concern for illness (lowered quality of life) has been the subject of substantial research (see e.g. Heritage and Robinson 2006; Mishler 1984). These divergent perspectives, though observable throughout the consultation where symptoms are topicalized, is brought to the fore first in the problem presentation phase, where the patient renders her own understanding of the illness, and in the subsequent diagnosis and treatment recommendation phases, where the GP's understanding, identification, and proposed solution of the problem are most clearly available (Heritage and Maynard 2006, p. 49, see also Frankel 2001, p. 85).

Primary care consultations, like all institutional communication, are goal-oriented. The goal, it has been argued, is treatment or cure (Robinson 2003; Stivers 2007). Frankel has argued that the physician's diagnosis is contingent upon both the initial problem statement and the questions and topics pursued by the doctor between the presentation of problem and the diagnosis delivery (Frankel 2001, p. 83). Other researchers similarly state that, essentially, diagnoses are responses to the patient's problem presentation (Robinson 2003, p. 50) and candidate diagnosis (Ijäs-Kallio et al. 2011). A symptom residue embodies a lack of fit in that the patient re-introduces symptoms first raised in the problem presentation that have not, come diagnosis or treatment recommendation, been sufficiently dealt with (Frankel 2001). As the analyses will show, this is not merely a matter of treatability.

Patients may, and do, raise and re-raise their understanding or information needs of a symptom throughout the course of the consultation (e.g. through offering lay or candidate diagnoses or by retelling their illness narrative). In this way, they successfully solicit physician evaluation. However, when such implicit or explicit information or evaluation requests are not met or addressed by the physician, the last place for the patient to influence the outcome of the consultation and address the symptom residue in search of a more sufficient solution is following the diagnosis or treatment recommendation. It is especially in these final phases that a mismatch may become apparent between 'the scope of the solution, the intervening discourse and the problem statement' (Frankel 2001, p. 98). A no-problem no-treatment evaluation (Stivers 2007), although this may be good news from a medical perspective in that a disease may have been ruled out, may signify bad news to the patient if it does not alleviate the life-world suffering she/he experiences but instead leaves the patient's symptom insufficiently addressed (Maynard and Frankel 2006, p. 278). However, because no communicative action is preferred following a diagnosis (Heath 1992, though see Peräkylä 1998, 2002) and because treatment recommendations have a tendency to be accepted, any extended response to diagnoses and any outcome other than acceptance of a recommendation is not preferred and treated by the physician as resistance (Stivers 2007). Introducing a residual symptom falls into this category, as it makes a response from the GP relevant, thereby opening a new sequence and halting the progression towards closure of the consultation. In many ways, symptom residue sequences then resemble what others have described as resistance. Stivers, for example, specifically mentions questions about symptoms as a form of resistance (Stivers 2007). However, symptom residue has not been investigated on its own, nor has the successful closure of these sequences been analysed. This chapter builds on insights on such resistance, but specifically seeks to understand the symptom residue variant and how it can, in these situations, be successfully navigated by the physician.

4.3 Data and Method

This chapter draws on a body of 43 audio- and/or video-recorded cases of talk on cough (a few are only one or the other due to technical difficulties). The cases are part of a larger corpus of 80 recordings of primary care consultations, primarily concerning respiratory tract infections with both antibiotic and non-antibiotic treatment outcomes. Some of the consultations in the present sub-collection are revisits because of persisting cough. Coughing itself as a communicative resource is not included except where it occurs along with talk of cough.

When initiated by the patient, talk on cough is overwhelmingly introduced during the problem presentation phase, either as the primary presenting concern (21 cases) or as part of a symptom conglomerate (11 cases). This shows that cough, in itself or in conjunction with other symptoms is, for the patients, doctorable that is, 'worthy of medical attention' (Heritage and Robinson 2006, p. 58). In another seven of the cases, GPs initiate talk on cough (in the remaining four cases, it is unclear who has initiated the talk, as the GP proceeds from information in the medical record which may have been either solicited or volunteered). Doctor-initiated talk on cough overwhelmingly occurs during, and helps constitute, the history-taking phase. Once talk on cough has been initiated, it is typically followed up either by probing questions from the GP and/or volunteered extra information from the patient.

Talk on cough occurs throughout the consultation, such that further insight is generated into how this symptom is understood by both patient and GP. This article focuses on symptom residue sequences. These are sequences where cough or its accompanying symptoms are re-introduced after a diagnosis. The sequences can take place online, during the physical examination or after the conclusion of the examination (physical or para-clinical) or treatment recommendation. Although originally used in relation to major illnesses, symptom residue is also an issue when minor illnesses and 'routine acute problems' such as the cold are discussed (Heritage and Robinson 2006 p. 50). Sequences of symptom residue are discerned from the related phenomena of additional symptoms (Nielsen 2012) and unmet concerns (Heritage et al. 2007). The basic criterion is that the symptom must be re-introduced, that is, it must have been mentioned during the initial problem presentation. The cases analysed in this chapter have been selected for their clarity and are representative of three most common symptom residue concerns, namely treatability, duration, and cause.

To analyse the symptom residue sequences, this article uses Conversation Analysis (CA). By analysing video recordings and detailed transcriptions of these recordings, CA allows for a step-by-step exploration of how each participant's utterance in a given communicative context (here, the consultation) affects and is affected by the other participants' turns-at-talk. Using this method enables the analysis of sequences of symptom residue as a co-constructed activity. For a key to the transcription symbols, see Nielsen (2018, Chap. 2).

4.4 Introducing and Responding to the Symptom Residue

When patients introduce a symptom residue, they primarily refer to specific aspects of the symptom experience: its treatability, its duration, or its cause (in some cases several of these). As the following analyses show, the response must be tailored to the aspects made relevant by the patient in order to sufficiently address the symptom residue. Due to space constraints, the full turn-by-turn resolution of the symptom residue will be included only in Example 3.

4.4.1 Treatability

At the beginning of the consultation, the patient in the excerpt has complained of cough and highlighted as primary concern the accompanying sleeplessness (caused by muscular, cough-related pain). In the excerpt below, based on the examination results and a rapid infection test, the GP rules out the cough as a sign of a problematic, bacterial infection.

Ex. 1 (06:49-07:19)

```
01   DOC:    ↑yes: (0.3) den var meget ↑LAV,
             yes(0.3) that was very ↑LOW,
02           (0.5)
03   DOC:    det tyder på at (.) det ikke er nogen bak↑terieinfektion som du ↓har.
             that suggests that what you have is not a bacterial infection
04           (0.2)
05   DOC:    men at det er en ↓virus.
             but that it is a virus
06   PAT:    (1.0)((lille nik))
             (1.0)((small nod))
07   DOC:    æ: og det betyder at antibiotika ikke vil (.) hjælpe dig.
             e: and that means that antibiotics will not help you
08   PAT:    ja.
             yes
09           (0.2)
10   DOC:    så:: det du kan ↑gøre det er de: almindelige (.) pleje sig ↑selv (.) ting,
             so what you can do is the usual take care of yourself stuff
11           som a::t (.) spise (.) ↓godt (.) sove  hvile,
             such as eat well sleep rest
12           (0.2)
13   PAT:    ja,
             yes
14   DOC:    så vil det blive bedre af sig selv.
             then it will get better on its own
15           (.)
16   PAT:    °↓okay.°.
             °↓okay.°
17   DOC:    [^yes,
             [^yes,
18   PAT:    [(k-)
             [(c-)
19   PAT:->  men Panodiler så jeg kan sove om natten det virker bare ikke,=
             but Panodil so I can sleep at night it just doesn´t work
20           =[altså så: æ:
             =[(ADV) so: e:
21   DOC:     [nej?
              [no?
22           er det sådan at du ligger v- oppe og hoster hele natten elle:r,
             are you lying awake and coughing all night or
```

Together with a prior diagnosis of the pain as muscular (no treatment recommendation, data not shown), the GP's no-problem no-treatment evaluation (l.1–5) provides both an explanation for the symptom (muscle pain) and an assertive diagnosis (virus). It is also used to account for the ruling out of a more serious diagnosis (bacterial infection) and antibiotic treatment. Finally, it concludes with an instruction to the patient of what he can do (next action step, l.10–11) and a prognosis of recovery (l.14).

The patient's responses, a delayed and minimal token agreement (l.13) and a soft 'okay' (l.16), are treated by the GP as acceptance with a 'yes' (l.17), which is simultaneously hearable as a possible move towards closure of the consultation (Schegloff and Sacks 1973). However, although initially aligning with the physician's recommendation, the patient uses this 'okay' as a transition into the introduction of the symptom residue.

While Maynard and Frankel (2006) find that the symptom residue stands in the way of the patient agreeing with the assessment of the good news, in the case here the patient does produce such agreeing assessments. However, the assessments function primarily as token agreements (or agreements on a partial solution), allowing a transition into the introduction of the symptom residue. With a but-prefaced objection that marks what follows as counter to this agreement—this patient, in overlap with the 'yes', resists the recommendation as insufficient, as he produces a symptom residue mention (l.19–20).

Part of this resistance may be due to the fact that the recommendation for a next action step as well as the prognosis (l.10, 11, and 14) is general, unspecific, and to some extent minimizes the problem (Stivers 2007). In the next turn, the patient specifically takes issue with the (now residual) symptom left unacknowledged (indeed, noticeably so: the GP recommends 'sleep' and 'rest' (l.11)), that the patient's concern is precisely lack of sleep due to cough-related back pain. This lifeworld problem, which the patient himself, in his presentation, has labelled 'the most annoying thing' (data not shown) though not a disease, is the symptom residue which the patient treats as still unresolved, even if not unexplained. Built into his turn is a specification.

He seeks pain relief, which he has unsuccessfully attempted to provide on his own (l.19).

With the discourse marker ‘so’ (l.20), the patient projects an unstated upshot, anticipating a solution-oriented response which invites the GP to introduce this due action (Raymond 2004, p. 190) and places the responsibility for providing a remedy with her. The GP, in response, re-enters the symptom exploration (l.22, followed by several other questions concerning the problem [data not shown]). Although the GP is the one introducing cough here, the patient, at the beginning of the consultation, has complained about pain and sleeplessness, and this has been expressly linked to cough. Thus, this link has already been established by both parties, and the patient’s mention of pain is hearable as a cough-related symptom residue even before the GP makes her understanding of this explicit. As a result of this symptom residue sequence, a remedy, another over-the-counter pain remedy, is eventually agreed upon and the consultation closed.

In other cases of symptom residue, treatability does not seem to be the issue. Instead, fear of a more serious diagnosis, fuelled by a lack of knowledge of normal prognosis (duration and/or course of the illness) or cause of accompanying symptoms, may be the reason. To successfully address this type of symptom residue, information addressing these aspects must been provided.

4.4.2 Duration

The patient, a child, is brought in by his mother. The symptom presentation centres on a cough which has persisted for four weeks even as other symptoms such as fever have subsided, except for an ear pain the night before the consultation. Upon lung auscultation, the GP makes a no-problem online commentary. A tentative viral diagnosis is made, but it is unclear whether this applies to the cough, the ear, or both. The GP has not informed the patient or parent of the course of a normal cough or how long it can be expected to last.

```
Ex. 2 (14:45-14:58)
01    DOC:     så men men det er inden for normalområdet=
               so but but it is within the normal range=
02             =det er ba:re (.) den er [lidt større
               =it is just (.) it is    [a bit bigger
03    MOM:                              [jaja °men det er fint, jh.a°
                                        [yes yes but that is fine, yes
04    DOC:     [og der er ikke nogen fa-
               [and there is no da-
05    MOM:-->  [det var mest den der ↓hoste jeg egentlig var bekymret for=
               [it was mostly that cough I was actually worried about=
06             =for jeg synes at den har stået på så længe ikke?
               =because I think it has persisted for so long no?
07    DOC:     ja,
               yes
08    MOM:     [men (.) (hvis det ikke er     )
               [but (.) (if it is not
09    PAT:     [((host)    [(host))
               [((cough))  [((cough))
10    DOC:     [m.         [der er mange som er forkøl[et nu.
               [m.         [there are many who have a cold now
11    MOM:                                            [ja
                                                      [yes
```

In response to the summary assessment, from which she may anticipate that the consultation is moving towards closure (Drew 2006, p. 441), the mother first fully accepts (l.3). This mirrors what we saw in Example 1, though expanded here. There is a token agreement and alignment, followed by the introduction of the symptom residue (l.5). As in Example 1 above, this overlaps with a turn by the GP which is hearable as closure-projecting, here an and-prefaced (Nevile 2006) ear-related statement.

Treating her turn as worth pursuing, the mother 'wins' the floor and reintroduces the cough for which she came to see the GP. This is initially formatted as an 'open' symptom residue introduction which does not specify what it is about the cough that causes concern (though marking the cough itself as previously mentioned and now reintroduced by the use of 'that' (l.5)). However, this is immediately specified in the subsequent account as the duration of the cough (l.6).

While the past tense in l.5 can be heard as orienting back to symptom duration as a matter of doctorability and using the duration as a legitimization of the visit (see Nielsen 2015), it also points forward to the symptom residue, the unaccounted for duration. By first aligning with the no-problem diagnosis, and then introducing the residue, the mother may be orienting to the delicacy of her action. Because the introduction makes an explanatory response relevant, opening up a new sequence and resisting the progression towards closure, it could be heard as the patient's questioning of the diagnosis. With the past tense, the use of 'mostly' and 'actually' (l.5) and the half-done retraction in l.8, she downgrades her epistemic stance and mitigates the resistance, thereby signalling respect for the GP's medical authority.

Due to space constraints, the entirety of the sequence cannot be shown here, but the GP engages by producing information that normalizes the specific duration mentioned by the mother. The sequence concludes with the GP restating the null-finding of the physical examination and ruling out a bacterial infection, which is now met with full acceptance. Nothing in this (nor the problem presentation) suggests a concern with treatability (such as a prescription for antibiotics) and in her response, the GP focuses on symptom explanation, not symptomatic treatment.

4.4.3 Cause

That the explanation of a symptom as much as *ruling out* a diagnosis may be another reason for raising a symptom residue is also clear from the following example, a revisit. The patient, a teenager accompanied by her mother, has made a candidate diagnosis of pneumonia. The patient had already been diagnosed with a viral throat infection by another physician but now feels her condition has worsened. Pain in the chest/sternum area is the main complaint, and the patient has confirmed coughing.

Ex. 3 (04:38-05:25)

```
01   DOC:    de:r er ikke spor at høre på lungerne.
             there is no trace of anything to hear on the lungs
02           (0.5)
03   PAT:    okay.
             okay
04   DOC:    så det e:r bare sådan en gang (.) god gang forkølelse.
             so it is just a case (.) good case of the cold
05   PAT:    (1.0) [okay fint nok.
             (1.0) [okay that´s fine.
06   DOC:          [så::
                   [so
07   MOM:    [så hjem at have varme [drikke,
             [so home and take hot drinks
08   DOC:    [ingen                 [ingen
             [no                    [no
09           ikke nogen lungebetændelse.
             not any pneumonia
             (0.5)
10   PAT:    >okay fint [nok.<
             >okay thats fine<
11   MOM: ->            [>nå men hvorfor gør det så ondt,=
                        [>well but why does it then hurt so=
12           =er det fordi hun har ↑hostet,<
             =is that because she has coughed
13   DOC:    ↓ja.
             ↓yes
14   MOM:    ↓okay.
             ↓okay.
15   DOC:    ↓ja .h  altså en lungebetændelse gør jo ikke ondt jo.
             ↓yes.h (ADV) a  pneumonia does (ADV) not hurt(ADV)
16   MOM:    nej [>men j- jeg ved det ikke fordi:
             no  [>but I- I don´t know because
17   DOC:        [nej.((nikker))
                 [no. ((nods))
18   MOM:    jeg kan ikke huske hvordan det var jeg selv havde det<
             i can´t remember how it was i myself felt<
19           da jeg havde °det nemlig°.
             when i had it you see
20   DOC:    man kan ikke mærke sine lunger men man kan mærke sine muskler omkring=
             you can´t feel your lungs but you can feel your muscles around=
21           =og man kan mærke jo også hvis det gør ondt oppe i halsen,
             =and you can also feel it (ADV) if it hurts up in the throat,
22   MOM:    okay.
             okay
```

```
23   DOC:   æ:: hvis man har hostet meget så får man jo o- også nemt nogle .hh
            eh: if you have coughed a lot, then you (ADV)a-  also easily get some .hh
24          nogle >symptomer der fra struben< h
            some >symptoms from the throat< h
25   MOM:   okay.
            okay
26   DOC:   men æ: men (.) lungerne er hElt rene at høre på så ↑ikke spor der.
            but eh but the lungs are completely clean to listen to so nothing at all
            there
27   PAT:   (0.5) ((nikker))
            (0.5) ((nods))
28   MOM:   [heldigt
            [fortunate
29   PAT:   [okay ja det er jeg godtnok glad for, ((smiler))
            [okay yes i am really happy about that ((smiles))
30   MOM:   ja.
            yes
31   DOC:   godt ((smiler))
            good ((smiles))
```

Similar to the patients in the previous examples, the mother and daughter align with the diagnostic evaluation (l.5, 7). But the no-treatment indicative diagnosis of 'no pneumonia' (l.9), which responds to the patient's initial candidate diagnosis (Ijäs-Kallio et al. 2011; Stivers 2007, p. 48), leaves unexplained the patient's main complaint: chest pain. With the patient´s acceptance of the negative diagnosis in l.10, the consultation could be proceeding towards closure. But here the mother interrupts to introduce the symptom residue. What is initially hearable as questioning the validity of the diagnosis (l.11) is in the next turn established as a question about the cause of the symptom (with the candidate explanation cough (l.12). This softens the introduction of the symptom residue from possibly accusatory to inquisitorial.

The GP confirms the explanation (l.13), but goes on to rule out the symptom as a possible sign of pneumonia (l.15), thereby orienting to the symptom residue mention as a form of resistance to the negative diagnosis. The (untranslatable) adverb '*jo*' (meaning 'as you/we know') indexes this knowledge (that the pain cannot be a sign of pneumonia) as already shared by the patient. This marks the question as inapposite, a morally transgressive action (see Heinemann et al. 2011 on the use of '*jo*'), which underscores that it is understood as resistance to the GP's diagnosis and epistemic authority. Subsequently, the mother aligns with the ruling out of the symptom of a sign of pneumonia (l.16), and the GP moves on to treat the matter as closed with his third turn 'no' (l.17). However, overlapping this, the mother (who may also at the same time be resisting that she has inappositely questioned the diagnosis) makes clear that this knowledge was not previously available to her (l.16–18). Thus, the GP's evaluation of the symptom is indirectly solicited again. In response, he then proceeds to affirmatively explain the cause of the symptom residue in more detail (l.20–24). Following this explanation, he reassures the patient by restating his examination null-finding, implicitly once more ruling out pneumonia, as well as any other serious illness (l.26). This time, the mother (and patient) explicitly treat this ruling out of the pain as a sign of pneumonia as good news and fully align with the physician's assessment (l.27–30), and the consultation moves into closure.

Through what resembles a local form of proof procedure, both parties treat the symptom residue sequence as sufficiently dealt with, so that a move towards closure can take place unimpeded.

4.5 Accounting for the Symptom Residue

While the symptom residue described by Maynard and Frankel (2006) remains because physicians do not know or are uncertain about the answer, the cases of cough indicate that here it seems to exist not because it *cannot* be accounted for (it subsequently is) but because, for whatever reason, it *has* not been accounted for.

Thus, the problem of symptom residue is not always a matter of uncertainty or irrationality. Instead, it seems to reflect a discrepancy about the understanding of a symptom: to the physician, the symptom is relevant for helping diagnose or exclude a possible disease (and treatment); for patients, the symptom is a problem in its own right because it results in lowered quality of life. This misalignment between perceptions of normality or abnormality of a symptom (Drew 2006, p. 444) and its differing significance to the physician and patient may stand in the way of closure of the consultation.

If, at the time of the diagnosis or treatment recommendation, the consultation has failed to deal sufficiently with a symptom of concern to the patient, the patient can resist the move towards closure and pursue the information through introducing the symptom residue.

In some symptom residue sequences, such as in Example 1 above, patients seem to desire a cure and will resist closure of the consultation until what they consider to be an adequate remedy is found. Such a remedy need not be, and indeed in these cases is not, an antibiotic prescription, but rather symptomatic, an affirmative, and specific next action step (Stivers 2007) that helps the patient manage the discomfort caused by the symptom. The symptom residue sequence gives the GP a (second) chance to offer these affirmative recommendations.

In other cases, however, treatability cannot be found to be the issue. Instead, patients are seen seeking information about normal illness duration and course (in Example 2), and explanations of the cause of the symptom (along with exclusion of a more serious disease), as in Example 3. These patients move towards sequence closure after receiving information, not after receiving treatment suggestions. What seems to resolve a symptom residue, then, is a response sufficiently fitted to it.

Whether it is information about symptom treatment, duration or cause, it is lack of information that leads to patient resistance to closure. Because the last occasion to introduce the symptom residue is after a diagnosis or treatment, this may be understood as a resistance to the non-antibiotic outcome. The patients mitigate this resistance by first aligning with the GP's diagnosis or recommendation and then accounting for their action (by specifying treatment, duration, or cause). In this way, they orient themselves to the delicacy of the matter while still introducing their concern. The GPs, instead of changing their recommendation and prescribing antibiotics in the face of this apparent resistance, re-engaged with the symptom and treated it not as pressure for antibiotics but as a need for more nuanced information, which was confirmed by the local proof procedure. This allowed the physicians to address the symptom residue without changing their diagnosis or recommendation. In addition, by re-engaging, the GPs may have gained insights into the patients' needs for information, thus allowing a more shared understanding of symptoms.

4.6 Resistance Revisited

Introducing a symptom residue does not necessarily equal resistance to the fact that a diagnosis or treatment recommendation does not project (antibiotic) treatment. In the present collection, even patients who are already in antibiotic treatment resist diagnoses or prognoses. When it becomes clear that the consultation may end with a diagnosis or treatment recommendation that does not sufficiently address the patient's initial concern, symptom residue is introduced. If the GP re-engages with a symptom presentation and tailors the response to the life-world concerns of the patient, not only to a medical assessment that rules out antibiotics or antibiotic implicative diagnosis (though they also do this), the patients are reassured and the consultation can close.

If GPs focus narrowly on the medical interpretation of symptoms, seeking to rule out diseases (and, as a consequence, prescription treatment), the patient may remain reluctant to let the consultation draw to a close because the symptom residue has not been managed. One alternative strategy for the GP to reach closure might have been to insufficiently address the patient's concern, which could result in re-consultations for the same or similar problems, increasing the risk of unnecessary antibiotics. Another strategy might have been to offer antibiotic treatment in the ongoing consultation as a way to close it. Both strategies, however, increase the risk of antibiotic resistance.

In the face of this perceived pressure, the GPs in this dataset have shown themselves to be attentive to the voiced needs and concerns of their patients. They successfully manage to bridge the discrepancy by providing a response tailored to patients' needs whether it be symptom treatment, explanation, or duration prognosis. Although they do occasionally treat the patients' ostensible diagnostic resistance as pressure for antibiotics (something also found by Stivers 2007), the GPs nonetheless overwhelmingly navigate the symptom residue sequences without offering this option, thereby reducing the overall risk of antibiotic resistance. GPs' willingness to engage with what can be perceived as patients' implicit (or explicit, see Nielsen 2018, Chap. 2) demands for antibiotics may be part of the explanation for the relatively low level of antimicrobial resistance in Denmark. Other explanations are addressed in the following chapters.

References

Beach, W. A., Easter, D. W., Good, J. S., & Pigeron, E. (2005). Disclosing and responding to cancer "fears" during oncology interviews. *Social Science & Medicine, 60*, 893–910. https://doi.org/10.1016/j.socscimed.2004.06.031

Cals, J. W., Hood, K., Aaftink, N., Hopstaken, R. M., Francis, N. A., Dinant, G. J., & Butler, C. C. (2009). Predictors of patient-initiated reconsultation for lower respiratory tract infections in general practice. *British Journal of General Practice, 59*, 761–764. https://doi.org/10.3399/bjgp09X472656

Drew, P. (2006). Misalignments in“after-hours” calls to a British GP's practice: A study in telephone medicine. *Studies in Interactional Sociolinguistics, 20*, 416.

Frankel, R. M. (2001). Clinical care and conversational contingencies: The role of patients' self-diagnosis in medical encounters. *Text, 21*, 83–11.

Heath, C. (1992). The delivery and reception of diagnosis in the general practice consultation. In P. Drew & J. Heritage (Eds.), *Talk at work, interaction in institutional settings*. Cambridge: Cambridge University Press.

Heinemann, T., Lindström, A., & Steensig, J. (2011). Addressing epistemic incongruence in question–answer sequences through the use of epistemic adverbs. In T. Stivers, L. Mondada, & J. Steensig (Eds.), *The morality of knowledge in conversation* (pp. 107–130). Cambridge: Cambridge University Press. https://doi.org/10.1017/CBO9780511921674.006

Heritage, J., & Maynard, D. W. (Eds.). (2006). *Communication in medical care: Interaction between primary care physicians and patients*. Cambridge: Cambridge University Press.

Heritage, J., & Robinson, J. D. (2006). The structure of patients' presenting concerns: Physicians' opening questions. *Health Communication, 19*, 89–102. https://doi.org/10.1207/s15327027hc1902_1

Heritage, J., Robinson, J. D., Elliott, M. N., Beckett, M., & Wilkes, M. (2007). Reducing patients' unmet concerns in primary care: The difference one word can make. *Journal of General Internal Medicine, 22*(10), 1429–1433. https://doi.org/10.1007/s11606-007-0279-0

Ijäs-Kallio, T., Ruusuvuori, J., & Peräkylä, A. (2011). Patient involvement in problem presentation and diagnosis delivery in primary care. *Communication & Medicine, 7*. https://doi.org/10.1558/cam.v7i2.131

Mangione-Smith, R., Elliott, M. N., Stivers, T., McDonald, L. L., & Heritage, J. (2006). Ruling out the need for antibiotics: Are we sending the right message? *Archives of Pediatrics & Adolescent Medicine, 160*, 945–952.

Maynard, D. W., & Frankel, R. M. (2006). On diagnostic rationality: Bad news, good news, and the symptom residue. In J. Heritage & D. W. Maynard (Eds.), *Communication in medical care* (pp. 248–278). Cambridge: Cambridge University Press.

Mishler, E. G. (1984). *The discourse of medicine: The dialectics of medical interviews*. Norwood, NJ: Ablex. pp. Xii, n.d.

Nevile, M. (2006). Making sequentiality salient: And-prefacing in the talk of airline pilots. *Discourse Studies, 8*(2), 279–302.

Nielsen, S. B. (2012). Patient initiated presentations of additional concerns. *Discourse Studies, 14*, 549–565.

Nielsen, S. B. (2015). "And how long have you been sick?": The discursive construction of symptom duration during acute general practice visits and its implications for "doctorability." *Time & Society*. https://doi.org/10.1177/0961463X15609808.

Nielsen, S. B. (2018). Dealing with explicit patient demands for antibiotics in a clinical setting. In C. S. Jensen, S. B. Nielsen, & L. Fynbo (Eds.), *Risking antimicrobial resistance* (pp. 61–77). Cham, Switzerland: Palgrave Macmillan.

Peräkylä, A. (1998). Authority and accountability: The delivery of diagnosis in primary health care. *Social Psychology Quarterly, 61*(4), 301–320.

Peräkylä, A. (2002). Agency and authority: Extended responses to diagnostic statements in primary care encounters. *Research on Language & Social Interaction, 35*, 219–247. https://doi.org/10.1207/S15327973RLSI3502_5

Raymond, G. (2004). Prompting action: The stand-alone "So" in ordinary conversation. *Research on Language & Social Interaction, 37*, 185–218. https://doi.org/10.1207/s15327973rlsi3702_4

Robinson, J. D. (2003). An interactional structure of medical activities during acute visits and its implications for patients' participation. *Health Communication, 15*, 27–59. https://doi.org/10.1207/S15327027HC1501_2

Schegloff, E. A., & Sacks, H. (1973). Opening up closings. *Semiotica, 8*(4), 289–327.

Stivers, T. (2007). *Prescribing under pressure: Parent-physician conversations and antibiotics*. Oxford: Oxford University Press.

Wigton, R. S., Darr, C. A., Corbett, K. K., Nickol, D. R., & Gonzales, R. (2008). How do community practitioners decide whether to prescribe antibiotics for acute respiratory tract infections? *Journal of General Internal Medicine, 23*, 1615–1620. https://doi.org/10.1007/s11606-008-0707-9

5

'To Prescribe or Not to Prescribe' is Not the Only Question: Physician Attitudes Towards Antibiotics and Prescription Practices in Spain

Sandi Michele de Oliveira, Nieves Hernández-Flores, and Vanesa Rodríguez-Tembrás

5.1 Introduction: Rationale for the Study and Current Situation in Spain

Antimicrobial resistance (AMR) and the risk to the health of the population has long been a concern in Spain, where tracking of antibiotic use dates back to at least the 1960s. The earliest comparison of Spanish and Danish data on antibiotic consumption and AMR we found was a study by Baquero Mochales et al. (1995, p. 449), which found that in the period 1966–1976, antibiotic consumption in Spain was four times

S. M. de Oliveira (✉) • N. Hernández-Flores
Department of English, Germanic and Romance Studies,
University of Copenhagen, Copenhagen, Denmark
e-mail: smo@hum.ku.dk; nhf@hum.ku.dk

V. Rodríguez-Tembrás
Department of Romance Languages, Institute for Translation and Interpretation, University of Heidelberg, Heidelberg, Germany
e-mail: vanesa.rodriguez@iued.uni-heidelberg.de

C. S. Jensen et al. (eds.), *Risking Antimicrobial Resistance*,
https://doi.org/10.1007/978-3-319-90656-0_5

higher as measured by the Daily Defined Dose (31 DDD/1000 inhabitants/day) than in Denmark. While the gap has narrowed significantly since that period, Spain continues to be one of the largest consumers of antibiotics in Europe and Denmark among the lowest, with 2015 rates found to be 22.2 DDD/1000 for Spain and 16.1 DDD/1000 for Denmark (The European Centre for Disease Prevention and Control; ECDPC 2015).

In the discussion of AMR, physicians' antibiotic prescription practices, particularly those in primary care (GPs) are at the heart of research initiatives. Examples of such studies are those by Llor and Bjerrum (2014) and Costelloe et al. (2010) focusing on over-prescription by GPs leading to overuse and imprudent prescription behaviours. Despite the fact that GPs account for more than 80 per cent of antibiotics prescribed in Spain (Gonzalez-Gonzalez et al. 2015: 2) and evidence shows that reducing 'inappropriate' prescriptions can lower both consumption and AMR, a review of the literature reveals that GPs are not the only actors in the antibiotic acquisition process. Others play a significant role in the continued overconsumption of antibiotics.

Among the other actors are secondary care health services. Álvarez Lerma et al. (2010) make an argument for assessing secondary care separately from primary care, as they find that antibiotic prescriptions in hospital and emergency care are justified differently than those in primary care. Cisneros et al. (2010, p. 29) claim that as many as 50 per cent of hospital prescriptions are 'unnecessary or inappropriate', with the study participants offering no consensus regarding how to improve the situation (Cisneros et al. 2010, p. 30). González-Castillo et al. (2013), examining emergency care practices, found a controversy regarding the best time to initiate antibiotic treatments when treating infectious diseases; they suggest that it would be 'common sense' for doctors to prescribe antibiotics preventatively (González-Castillo et al. 2013, p. 178).

While only physicians can prescribe antibiotics, patients can acquire and consume antibiotics through other means in Spain. In fact, the patient is actually a critical actor in understanding rational antibiotic use. This applies to two different types of situations, both of which lay outside the direct control of GPs. On one hand, patients may engage in self-medication with antibiotics, or they may choose not to take the medication prescribed. According to a survey reported in Eurobarometer (2013), self-medication among Spanish patients accounted for eight per cent of all antibiotic use, higher than the European average of five per cent. Of this Spanish group of eight per cent, half obtained antibiotics without prescription and half had saved medication from an earlier prescription (Eurobarometer 2013, p. 12). Recent studies suggest that as many as 42 per cent of households have at least one package of antibiotics and 30 per cent have retained antibiotics from a previous prescription, with 67 per cent of the respondents believing that there was no problem with saving antibiotics for later use (RSS 2017).

In spite of strict controls governing antibiotic distribution in pharmacies, some pharmacists continue to be susceptible to patients' requests for antibiotics without a prescription. Salar (2006, p. 267) found that 18.9 per cent of all requests for antibiotics were made without a prescription. Llor and Cots (2009), in a study of actors who simulated various medical problems at 197 pharmacies in northeast Spain, including asking for an antibiotic without a prescription, found that in 45 per cent of the pharmacies simulations were successful and the actors obtained antibiotics. Appeals based on symptoms are not the only tactic that patients may use: another factor is the familiarity between the pharmacist and the patient/consumer. Caamaño Isorna et al. conducted a study of the 166 pharmacies in one of Spain's regions. Nearly all (163) responded to a questionnaire, self-reporting on whether they provided antibiotics to their customers without a prescription. Pharmacists in the aggregate demanded prescriptions of their regular clients 34 per cent of the time, but fully 59 per cent of the time when asked by non-regular or first-time clients (Caamaño Isorna et al. 2004, p. 407).

Perspectives on prescription practices, physician behaviour, antibiotics, AMR, and the availability of medication without prescription through pharmacies are addressed at length in the medical literature. For the most part, the methodology chosen has been quantitative in nature, making possible the analysis of the dimension and extension of findings that the researchers have already defined. However, this type of inquiry does not generally permit a detailed explanation of the factors analysed, nor does it allow for the identification of new factors that may influence the overall interpretation of the situation. A study by Gonzalez-Gonzalez et al. (2015) includes a qualitative focus, examining various factors that could influence the doctor when prescribing antibiotics. Their qualitative approach thus adds a broader, more complex dimension to the statistical studies. For these reasons, Gonzalez-Gonzalez et al. constitutes a valuable study for examining attitudes and practices related to antibiotics and AMR.

The design of the Gonzalez-Gonzalez et al. study had three phases. In the first phase, four physician focus groups were established. The topics were (a) professional knowledge on antibiotics and AMR; (b) physicians' *fear* of complications if symptoms are left untreated; (c) physicians' attribution of responsibility to *external factors*, such as the continued availability of antibiotics without prescription; and (d) physicians' attribution of importance to satisfying patients' desires, demands, or expectations (referred to as '*complacencia*' (Gonzalez-Gonzalez 2015, p. 3; López-Vázquez 2015, p. 104). As a side note, we have reverted to the original Spanish term in this chapter, as 'complacency' in English often refers to unaware self-satisfaction. In the second phase of the research, based on the analysis of the focal group data, 1428 GPs in Galicia, one of the regions of our study, completed an 11-statement questionnaire. In the third phase, the researchers used the questionnaire data to correlate physicians' attitudes with their actual prescription practices.

One aim of our study is to provide contextual knowledge about the decision-making process that physicians use to prescribe. In contrast to the Gonzalez-Gonzalez et al. study, we define the categories of analysis based on the physician interviews. In this way, we discover the categories that doctors use not only to report their attitudes and behaviour, but also to justify them. We view the acquisition and use of antibiotics in Spain as a complex system: the physician is not the only relevant actor, and the curative function of antibiotics is not the only rationale driving prescription practices, the patient plays a critical role in achieving rational antibiotic use and antibiotic consumption is possible through means other than prescription. This complexity is evident in the first part of our chapter title 'To prescribe or not to prescribe is not the only question'. Our study analyses physician perspectives as obtained through qualitative interviews, thus bringing to light a broad range of relevant factors that can influence antibiotic use. Rather than collapsing analytical categories to achieve better statistical results, we seek here to explore the breadth of information provided. We do so by emphasizing the communicative and social context in which decisions are made. The choice to focus on physicians may seem counter-intuitive in light of our stated purpose to understand the system as a whole. However, as only physicians who have the authority to prescribe antibiotics, it is critical to have a thorough understanding of their decision-making processes under pressure—from official quarters and from patients.

In this chapter, we begin by examining physician opinions and attitudes regarding antibiotics, including preventative uses, AMR, and patients' views on taking medication. Our second focus is on the primary care consultation and the considerations that may arise which might influence the physician to prescribe an antibiotic. Such considerations may be professional or clinical in nature, but they are often subject to social, personal, cultural, and communicative influences, such as the argumentative strategies used by patients to obtain or reject medication. Our third focus is on the role of actors and institutions outside primary care, notably those that the physicians interviewed claimed would exert pressure toward greater antibiotic use (hospitals, private doctors, patient actions, and pharmacies).

5.2 Methodology

This study is based on physician interviews conducted in Spain in 2014. The interviews are extracted from two corpora that also include audiotapes of primary care, paediatric and emergency care consultations, patient questionnaires, as well as interviews with health administrators and researchers (Oliveira and Hernández-Flores 2014a, b). This section presents an overview of the participants and the interview questions.

5.2.1 Participants

The 25 physicians interviewed for this study include 15 GPs (indicated as GP1–GP15) and 10 geriatric specialists (labeled as GE1–GE10).

Table 5.1 Areas covered in all interviews

General topics	Information sought
Physician information	Age, gender, medical specialization, years as practicing doctor, years in the clinic, overall characterization of the patients, and average time spent consulting with each patient.
Structure of consultations	Use of time in the consultation, constraints on the doctor due to time, and view of patients' degree of trust in the doctor.
Unfolding communication between the doctor and patient	Patients' preparation for the consultation, if any; passive versus active patients; and views on the importance of trust between doctors and patients (and how it is manifest).
Participation of patient in the decision-making process	Opinions on inclusion of the patient in the treatment decision-making process and techniques for achieving it.
Use of antibiotics	Symptoms that indicate a need for antibiotics, ways of handling ambiguous cases, patient requests for more or fewer antibiotics and related argumentation strategies, and arguments used by doctors to withhold antibiotic prescriptions.

Interviews ranged from 15 to 80 minutes, depending on the work constraints of each physician.

In our semi-structured interviews, after obtaining basic information on each participant's age and professional background, we centred on four main topics (see Table 5.1). Our approach was ethnographic in nature: we allowed the participants the freedom to develop their answers as they saw fit and adjusted our questioning priorities according to the time available for the interview. The following table indicates questions asked of all participants relevant to the focus of this chapter.

5.3 Analysis of Interview Data

Discourse analysis of the interviews makes it clear that physicians are (a) aware of over-prescription as a factor in the increase of AMR and (b) aware of 'abuses' in the system (11 physicians cited AMR without prompting). Even so, eight of the 25 physicians claimed that the prescription of antibiotics for other than clinically appropriate reasons is the exception rather than the norm, and they expect to base their decision to prescribe on a clinical diagnosis. These statements represent the underlying mindset of the physicians who, along with the health administration's established prescription policies, form the baseline for action by the physician. Moreover, there exists an established protocol for handling situations of doubt in primary care consultations; namely, to ask the patient to return in three days if symptoms worsen (mentioned by 11 of the 25 physicians).

Underlying the rationales used by physicians to prescribe antibiotics for reasons other than unambiguous clinical symptoms is the desire to provide preventative care. With preventative care viewed as potentially unnecessary and a contributor to the development of AMR, some physicians mitigate its negative connotation, speaking of 'acceptable' versus 'non-acceptable' prevention. Two doctors use special terms to distinguish between the two: GE3 uses the terms 'primary' and 'secondary' prevention, the latter being acceptable, while GP2 refers to 'precaution' and 'prevention', the former being acceptable and GE6 uses a war metaphor to express acceptable prevention: 'act promptly when you see the enemy'. The primary justification of preventative prescriptions is an assessment of the general strength of the patient and ability to ward off potential infection, a finding in line with González-Castillo et al.'s (2013) commonsense approach to prescription.

In the next sub-section, we present situations that physicians report having arisen during a GP consultation that affect the physician's decision to prescribe antibiotics. In the second sub-section, we focus on physician-reported situations occurring outside the primary care consultation context that might lead to greater use of antibiotics, as well as the individuals and institutions that aid them in this effort.

5.3.1 Reported Practices within the GP Consultation

Physicians cited time pressures as a major factor in handling patients whose diagnosis is not clear. As consultations in Spain are ostensibly limited to an average of seven minutes, GPs stated that unless they find clear reasons for prescribing an antibiotic, they would ask the patient to return in three days for an updated evaluation, as mentioned above.

Despite this policy, GPs make exceptions based on a variety of circumstances; they cited three types of rationales for exceptions. One is of a medical nature: the physician may decide to prescribe because the clinical diagnosis is ambiguous (GP4, GP6, GP11, and GP12) or due to the patient's general health and previous illnesses (GP4, GP5, GP6, GP7, and GP12). In these cases, the GP weighs the risk of complications due to previous or chronic illnesses, advanced age, or other factors.

Another rationale is of a social and communicative nature: of the 21 physicians who commented on patient pressure to prescribe (or withhold a prescription), 11 said they had encountered cases of patients insisting on medication. Of these, however, only five revealed that they had given into pressure (GP3, GP4, GP11, GP12, and GE5), after becoming, in their words, 'exhausted' due to repeated calls for medication. In contrast, ten physicians stated that their patients have not applied this type of pressure.

The third reason for prescribing medication arises from a patient's difficulty in returning within the timeframe the doctor has set. The consultation's proximity to a weekend or vacation period might lead the doctor to write a 'preventative prescription' for use only if symptoms worsen (GP3 and GP12). Another consideration is the profession of the patient, such as that of lorry driver, whose normal job responsibilities require long or frequent trips away from the area (GP3 and GP12). Physicians use a similar reasoning if a patient lives far from the health centre and has limited options for transportation (GP2, GP3, and GP9).

As indicated above, doctor–patient communication in the consultation is a key factor in making medical decisions, and all physicians highlighted communication when asked about the importance of involving the patient in the treatment decision-making process: if the patient is not an active partner in the discussion, the treatment may not be carried out appropriately. Physicians report that patients who agree to treatment without antibiotics do so because they trust their doctor. Moreover, patients have an ever-increasing awareness of risks associated with overprescription due to health education, institutional initiatives, and discussion in the media.

Despite the physicians' statement that most patients accept their advice, many recounted argumentative strategies used by patients to obtain antibiotics when a prescription is not forthcoming. One type of patient argument presented was that the patients claimed to know someone who had similar symptoms and was treated and cured with antibiotics (GP4, GP5, GP6, GP7, GE5, and GE8). Other doctors mentioned that patients sometimes claim that they cannot stay home from work and believe that an antibiotic will help them get back on their feet quickly (GP3 and GP12). Other physicians cite patients who argue that a friend or family member (a layperson) suggested they might need an antibiotic (GP2 and GP3). Finally, a very few doctors report that patients threaten to go elsewhere if the GP does not prescribe an antibiotic (GP1 and GP6).

Twelve of the 25 physicians in our study affirmed that among patients questioning the doctor's decision to prescribe (or not), the likelihood was greater that patients would ask for more rather than less medication, for the reasons mentioned above. However, eight of the 25 physicians had patients wishing not to take medication. One reason they provide is that the patients had read about the dangers of side-effects in medication or antibiotics in general (D12 and D19). Another case was that of patients with chronic illnesses who said they wished to reduce the amount of their medication overall (GP3, GE2, and GE4). In these cases, the concern of the doctor is that these patients may receive the prescription but not actually take the medication or, alternatively, they may stop taking the medication when they begin to feel better.

5.3.2 Practices Outside the GP Consultation

The foregoing strategies involve communication and actions that take place during the actual consultation. In this section, we consider some of the external factors that the physicians believe influence the patient's attitudes and behaviours regarding antibiotic use. Physicians in our study mentioned patients' consultation of private doctors and private medical centres as alternative recourses for patients seeking an antibiotic prescription (GP1, GP3, and GP6); physicians obtained this information from the patients themselves, who described the actions they took after consulting their GP.

Regarding antibiotic use in hospitals and including geriatric patients, many doctors stated that antibiotics are much more widely distributed in secondary care than in primary care (GP4, GP8, GE2, GE3, GE5, GE6, GE7, GE9, and GE10), corroborating findings by Álvarez Lerma et al. (2010). While geriatric doctors are no less aware of the relationship between overconsumption and antibiotic resistance than GPs, they tend to consider the overall health of the patient, her or his age, previous illnesses, previous hospital admittances and earlier over-prescription. One doctor said, semi-jokingly, 'at least antibiotic resistance is proof they are still alive' (GE6).

Among the rationales offered by geriatric doctors for prescribing antibiotics in situations that the legislation and policy may deem unnecessary or inappropriate were the following:

- Geriatric patients (aged 75 years and above) generally present more serious illnesses than those in primary care. If they have had to re-enter the hospital, their case is considered serious (GE4, GE6, and GE7);
- Antibiotics may result in a shorter hospital stay, with the patient taking the antibiotics home and following up with her or his GP (GE1, GE3, GE6, and GE7);
- Antibiotics can be a preventative measure when there are indications that the patient may develop an infection (GE1, GE3, GE4, GE5, and GE6).

Patient use of emergency care was another topic mentioned by GPs as an alternative source for prescriptions (GP2, GP3, GP4, GP5, and GP12); doctors reported patients having 'confessed' that they had gone to emergency care under certain specific circumstances:

- Greater likelihood of obtaining a prescription generally;
- Greater flexibility in hours, to avoid work schedule incompatibility;
- Urgent need for medication due to upcoming travel (work or vacation).

According to physicians, patients unsuccessful in obtaining a prescription view pharmacies as their last resort. Despite the legal controls regulating the access to antibiotics, financial sanctions and a new system of electronic prescriptions in most regions of Spain (e.g. 80 per cent of all prescriptions in Galicia were electronic by February 2016, according to Cano 2016), many pharmacists remain susceptible to arguments by patients, who now take on the role of demanding consumers. One physician said that her patients make comments such as 'You go to the pharmacy, tell him your symptoms, and he will give you something' or 'You tell him you will bring the prescription on another day and he'll give you the medicine' (GE10). These comments provide anecdotal corroboration of the Caamaño Isorna et al. study (2004; see above) showing pharmacists' preferential treatment for regular customers.

These facts show that independent of the patient's attitude and behaviour in the medical consultations, the patient plays an active role in the treatment process. Above, we discussed non-filling of prescriptions and incomplete treatment. Several physicians referred to incomplete treatments and the need to inform the patients of the associated risks of unfinished treatment (GP2, GP7, GP9, GE5, and GE6), further mentioning that many patients save unused antibiotics for later use by themselves or other family members.

5.4 Discussion: Prescription Practices and Beyond

This chapter has addressed the prescription and use of antibiotics in Spain in the context of Spain's relatively high percentage of antibiotic resistance compared to other European countries. Research conducted by physicians tends to focus on the quantitative analysis of physician *behaviour* and the factors that influence it. In contrast, our qualitative approach has examined antibiotic use as a system in which both medical and other factors (social, logistical, ethical, and cultural) come into play. All these factors influence the physicians' decision to prescribe antibiotics, as well as the patients' actions in acquiring or rejecting antibiotics, and then actually taking their prescribed medication.

Through the analysis of interviews with 25 Spanish physicians, we began by identifying attitudes towards and practices regarding the use of antibiotics. Here we found that these attitudes are in general agreement with official policies that consumption of antibiotics should be restricted to cases of necessity. We divided the interview data into two groups: (1) practices and the attitudes that govern them within the framework of the GP consultation and (2) factors which occur outside the direct control of the GP and might influence their prescription practices. In primary care consultations, the physician faces the dilemma set forth in the first part of this chapter's title, 'to prescribe or not to prescribe'. The physician knows the medical conditions and protocols under which prescription is appropriate, but it is in the context of the consultation that she or he makes the ultimate decision. This decision is made after assessing the patient's current medical condition and its severity, along with any medical history suggesting that an infection could have serious consequences for the patient's overall health. Prescribing under these conditions is associated with preventative care, and our data has enabled us to distinguish between prescription practices for curative versus preventative purposes. Physicians report that preventative prescriptions motivated for clinical reasons are acceptable medical practice, to the point that doctors explain and defend the scientific rationale underlying their decision, even employing new terms to counteract the negative connotation associated with 'prevention' as being unnecessary.

Along with clinical factors, we identified social and situational factors that can affect the decision to prescribe, such as the social or professional life of the patient, work constraints, travel, or an illness coinciding with the patient's vacation. In these cases, knowledge of and communication with the patient are fundamental in determining whether the situation warrants a preventative prescription, whether it be in primary or emergency care. If so, parameters of a social and cultural nature override the scientific criteria of the physician. However, the physicians themselves speak of 'treating the whole patient' and view this behaviour as part of what constitutes 'good medical practice'.

Consideration of social factors led us to the second part of the title, that the decision to prescribe based purely on medical assessment *is not the only question* when examining the issue of AMR. Institutional, social and psychosocial, cultural and communicative considerations also influence the decision. At the institutional level, there is no ambiguity regarding the structure and functioning of the health system in Spain, its organization, the responsibilities of different actors, and the professional roles they play relative to the distribution and use of antibiotics. However, under a variety of circumstances, patients can still obtain antibiotics without prescription.

Social expectations on the part of patients also attest to the importance of recognizing non-clinical factors that can arise and influence the negotiation of treatment. Among the factors mentioned in the interviews is the perception that a patient's familiarity with the doctor or pharmacist may give them an advantage in obtaining services or medicine; that 'service' implies meeting the needs of the patient, and that patients may expect the granting of personal favours, both elements of *complacencia.* These social expectations reveal what we might term as *flexibility* in the sociocultural environment, as opposed to 'cracks' or breakdowns in the system. In fact, these and other aspects of the Spanish cultural community play a definite role in determining a patient's likelihood of obtaining antibiotics in the absence of medical necessity.

In conclusion, this study has provided information and clarification on the beliefs of the Spanish doctors in our data corpus, as well as their values regarding practices both within and outside the GP consultation. The study has shown that adherence to protocol in the prescription of antibiotics is not the only factor determining whether antibiotics are prescribed. Contextual considerations of a medical nature as well as social, cultural, and institutional considerations also come into play in the acquisition and consumption of antibiotics. In this complex situation, the patient assumes principal importance, both in their communication with the GP as well as outside the primary care consultation. As the physicians themselves reveal other factors that they believe influence patient actions to seek (additional) medication or to abandon treatments prematurely, the natural next research step is to look towards the actor whose role in the treatment process has been under-analysed, if not overlooked, in the medical literature: the patient.

References

Álvarez Lerma, F., Sierra Camerino, R., Álvarez Rocha, L., & Rodríguez Colomo, O. (2010). Política de antibióticos en pacientes críticos. *Medicina intensiva, 34*(9), 600–608.

Baquero Mochales, F., Baraibar Castelló, R., Campos Marques, J., Dominguez Rodríguez, L., Garau Alemany, X., et al. (1995). Resistencia microbiana: ¿Qué hacer? *Revista Española de Salud Pública, 69*(6), 445–461.

Caamaño Isorna, F., Tomé-Otero, M., Takkouche, B., & Figueiras, A. (2004). Factors related with prescription requirement to dispense in Spain. *Pharmacoepidemiology and Drug Safety, 13*(6), 405–409.

Cano, M. (2016). Receta electrónica. *eyrieSalud.* [blog] 19 February 2016. Retrieved January 2017, from http://www.eyriesalud.com/2016/02/19/receta-electronica/

Cisneros, J. M., Ortiz-Leyba, C., Lepe, J. A., Obando, I., Conde, M., et al. (2010). Uso prudente de antibióticos y propuestas de mejora desde la medicina hospitalaria. *Enfermedades Infecciosas y Microbiología Clínica, 28*(Suppl. 4), 28–31.

Costelloe, C., Lovering, A., & Hay, A. D. (2010). Effect of antibiotic prescribing in primary care on antimicrobial resistance in individual patients: Systematic review and meta-analysis. *The British Medical Journal (thebmj), 340*, c2096.

European Centre for Disease Prevention and Control (ECDPC). (2015). Trend of the consumption of Antibacterials for Systemic Use (ATC group J01) in the community (primary care sector) in Spain, Denmark from 1997 to 2015. Retrieved January 2017, from http://ecdc.europa.eu/en/healthtopics/antimicrobial-resistance-and-consumption/antimicrobial-consumption/esac-net-database/Pages/trend-consumption-by-country.aspx

European Commission. Antimicrobial Resistance Report. (2013). *Antimicrobial resistance.* Special Eurobarometer 407. Retrieved January 2017, from https://ec.europa.eu/health/sites/health/files/antimicrobial_resistance/docs/ebs_407_en.pdf

González-Castillo, J., Candel, F. J., & Julián-Jiménez, A. (2013). Antibióticos y el factor tiempo en la infección en urgencias. *Enfermedades Infecciosas y Microbiología Clínica, 31*(3), 173–180.

Gonzalez-Gonzalez, C., López-Vázquez, P., Vázquez-Lago, J. M., Piñeiro-Lamas, M., Herdeiro, M. T., Arzamendi, P. C., et al. (2015). Effect of physicians' attitudes and knowledge on the quality of antibiotic prescription: A cohort study. *PLoS ONE, 10*(10), e0141820. Retrieved January 17, 2017. https://doi.org/10.1371/journal.pone.0141820.

Llor, C., & Bjerrum, L. (2014). Antimicrobial resistance: Risk associated with antibiotic overuse and initiatives to reduce the problem. *Therapeutic Advances in Drug Safety, 5*(6), 229–214.

Llor, C., & Cots, J. M. (2009). The sale of antibiotics without prescription in pharmacies in Catalonia, Spain. *Clinical Infectious Diseases, 48*(10), 1345–1349.

López Vázquez, P. M. (2015). *Influencia de las actitudes de los médicos en la utilización de antibióticos en Atención Primaria: un estudio de cohortes.* Doctoral dissertation (unpublished), Universidad de Santiago de Compostela.

Oliveira, S. M. de, & Hernández-Flores, N. (2014a). *Corpus médico de Castilla-La Mancha. UC-CARE Project on doctor-patient communication.* Corpus (unpublished), University of Copenhagen, Denmark.

Oliveira, S. M. de, & Hernández-Flores, N. (2014b). *Corpus de interacción médico-paciente de Galicia. UC-CARE Project on doctor-patient communication.* Corpus (unpublished), University of Copenhagen, Denmark.

Responsabilidad Social Sanitaria y Sociosanitaria (RSS). (2017). España se automedica: Una de cada tres personas consume antibióticos sin receta. 27 April 2017. Retrieved May 2017, from https://www.responsabilidadsociosanitaria.com/secciones/salud-sociedad/espana-se-automedica-uno-de-cada-tres-personas-consume-antibioticos-sin-receta-3276

Salar, L. (2006). *Estudio de la demanda de antibióticos sin receta en la oficina de farmacia. Papel del farmacéutico en la automedicación con antibióticos.* Doctoral dissertation, Universidad CEU Cardenal Herrera. Retrieved January 2017, from https://www.reap.es/docs/TesisLuisSalar.pdf

6

Governing the Consumption of Antimicrobials: The Danish Model for Using Antimicrobials in a Comparative Perspective

Carsten Strøby Jensen

6.1 Introduction

This chapter discusses how different governmental structures and regulative frameworks, at national and international levels, attempt to govern the consumption of antimicrobials in order to control the development of antimicrobial resistance (AMR). This chapter focuses on a case study of Denmark, analyzing how governmental structures influence the level of consumption of antimicrobials, both within the veterinary and the human sectors.

The point of departure for the focus on government regulations in this chapter is based on two observations. First, antimicrobial consumption differs very much from one country to another and that the national differences in consumption correlate significantly with levels of AMR (Aarestrup 1999; European Commission 2015). And second, compared to other countries, Denmark has a low level of antimicrobial consumption. This is the case within both the veterinary and the human sectors.

C. S. Jensen (✉)
Department of Sociology, University of Copenhagen, Copenhagen, Denmark
e-mail: csj@soc.ku.dk

C. S. Jensen et al. (eds.), *Risking Antimicrobial Resistance*,
https://doi.org/10.1007/978-3-319-90656-0_6

The relatively low level of Danish antimicrobial consumption concurs with a number of measures taken by government agencies during the past 20 years. In Denmark, reduction of antimicrobial consumption has for several years been high on the political agenda in order to reduce the spread of AMR (DANMAP 2016).

These two observations lead to the obvious question of whether Denmark's low level of antimicrobial consumption is tied to specific governmental and regulative initiatives at a national level. The term 'governmental structures' refers to different types of formal (or to a certain degree informal) regulations (e.g. legislation) initiated by national or international political authorities that attempt to affect the behavior of humans within the jurisdiction of the political authority. In the literature, governmental initiatives can be analyzed within a number of different theoretical perspectives. In this context, two theoretical perspectives frame the analysis of how governmental structures influence the level of antimicrobial consumption in Denmark. The first perspective relates to the collective action problem and the potential contradiction between the interests of the individuals and the interests of society as a whole. The collective action perspective is used to analyze why there is a need for governmental regulation of antimicrobial consumption. The second theoretical framework is based on principal–agent theory, which focuses on relations between a principal (e.g. a government) and an agent (e.g. user of antimicrobials). The principal–agent theory is widely used in organizational studies and political science and is discussed below in more detail.

Further in this chapter, Sect. 6.3 discusses the use of antimicrobials in a comparative perspective, presenting data from several countries. It also discusses the association between high antibiotic use and the development of AMR. Section 6.4 focuses specifically on Denmark, presenting the overall Danish governmental and regulative framework for using antibiotics. I argue that the comparatively low level of antibiotic resistance in Denmark is a result of the specific national legislation on antibiotic use. Most antimicrobials are used among the general practitioners, and the section analyzes the possibilities and problems tied to regulating the use of antimicrobials within the human sector. A part of the section focuses especially on the veterinary sector, and especially on the use of antimicrobials in relation to pig production. In Denmark, around 30 million swine are produced every year, and nearly one-third of the overall yearly consumption of antimicrobials in Denmark is used within this production. Nevertheless, the level of antimicrobial consumption per swine in Denmark is considerably lower than in other swine-breeding countries. This section describes how the use of antimicrobials is managed in Danish pig production. Finally, the concluding Sect. 6.5 discusses the applicability of the Danish experience in terms of international trends and possibilities for reducing AMR.

6.2 Principal–Agent Theory and the Collective Action Problem

Consumption of antimicrobials and the increasing levels of AMR can usefully be analyzed within what is called 'the collective action problem'. Within sociology, 'the collective action problem' describes situations where a group of individuals—if they act rationally—will perform certain actions that are not in the interests of the overall group. A given action may be rational when seen from the individuals' perspective but irrational when viewed from the overall society's perspective due to undesirable consequences. This situation describes the dilemma of antimicrobial consumption and AMR. Seen from the individual citizen's perspective, the use of antimicrobials is rational in the sense that it can be an effective weapon against infections and disease. At the same time, it is relatively harmless, easy to consume, and very cheap. Using antimicrobials is thus an attractive choice for the individual. Seen from the community's perspective, however, the widespread consumption of antimicrobials creates a risk of resistance (AMR). Increased AMR reduces the effectiveness of antimicrobials in situations where there might be life-threatening infections. Hence, there is a collective action problem.

In the organizational literature, governmental regulation is often presented as one of the options through which collective action problems can be managed. Governments and states acts as collective actors, frequently attempting to mediate between the interests of individuals/groups and the general interests of society. Governments regulate with the purpose of managing the collective interests of the populations under their control.

How governments deal with the collective interests of a population versus the interests of the individuals through different types of governmental initiatives can be analyzed within a principal–agent theoretical framework. Principal–agent theory analysis is widely used in organizational studies and within political science (Aulakh and Gencturk 2000; Elgie 2002). The focus of principal–agent theory is on how a given principal (e.g. a manager of a company or a government) governs the agents (e.g. staff members of a company or 'the population') in situations where the interests of the principals and the agents may diverge.

The principal–agent theory operates with three axioms. First, both the principal and the agent will try to act in a utility-maximizing way. They will act in a way that increases and satisfies their interests and utility. Second, the principal and the agent have different goals. They do not have common interests. The third axiom is that principals' and agents' access to information is asymmetrical. The agent has access to more information than the principal. This implies that the principal cannot be sure that the agent acts in line with the goals of the principals.

Further in this chapter, we will analyze which type of principal–agent relations are used by Danish public authorities to solve the collective action problems related to antibiotic consumption.

6.3 Consumption of Antimicrobials in a Comparative Perspective

Despite the fact that medical standards for using antimicrobials are very similar across states, actual consumption levels differ from country to country (and within countries). One specific and internationally recognized recommendation is that antimicrobials should only be used for bacterial infections and not for viruses. Antimicrobials have no effect against viruses. However, there are some estimates indicating that almost half of all global antimicrobial consumption among humans at the community level (outside hospitals) is used for coughs and colds, although antimicrobials have no medical effects on these illnesses (Gelband et al. 2015, p. 10).

Statistics of antimicrobial consumption can be divided into antimicrobials used for humans and antimicrobials used for livestock animals (but also increasingly for companion animals).

Generally, antimicrobials are used for humans to treat bacterial infections such as respiratory tract infections and urinary tract infections. However, they are also used for prophylactic purposes, in connection with hip replacement, heart transplantation, or other post-operative care.

Among livestock animals, antimicrobials are also used to combat different types of infections in wounds, organs or on the skin. Chickens, swine, cattle, and other livestock receive antimicrobials on a regular basis in connection with modern farming, where large herds of animals live together in a limited space. However, antimicrobials are also used as growth promoters. Antimicrobials increase the growth of livestock animals and, since the 1950s, have been used regularly as growth promoters in a number of countries. This practice has been prohibited in the European Union (EU) (from 2005) and other countries due to the risk of AMR. In the USA, however, antimicrobials are still used as growth promoters.

6.3.1 Human Consumption

As mentioned above, it is possible to observe differences in the level of consumption of antimicrobials between countries. This can be seen in Table 6.1, which shows the defined daily dose (DDD—defined daily dose per 1000 inhabitants/day) of antimicrobials among humans in a selected group of OECD countries. The DDD describes the assumed

Table 6.1 Consumption of antimicrobials in selected OECD countries, 2013, expressed as DDD per 1000 inhabitants and per day

Chile	9.4
Germany	15.8
Korea	16.2
Denmark	16.4
OECD-average (29)	20.7
UK	21.7
Australia	22.8
Italy	28.6
France	30.1
Greece	32.2
Turkey	42.2

Source: OECD (2015, p. 138)

average maintenance dose per day for a drug used for its main indication in adults. The use of the DDD index makes it possible to identify and compare antibiotic consumption per capita in different countries.

Variations in the use of antimicrobials in the human sector are quite considerable among the OECD countries. In 2013, the average DDD per 1000 inhabitants in OECD countries was 20.7 DDD. However, the level of use among the OECD countries varied by a factor of four, from 9.4 DDD in Chile to a high value of 42.2 DDD in Turkey.

A corresponding difference in the consumption of the so-called 'critical' types of antimicrobials can also be observed. Critical types of antimicrobials are regarded as critical due to their importance in human medicine (WHO 2017). They are, for example, quinolones and cephalosporins, for which it is recommended that they be used only when other types of antimicrobials have no effect.

A 16-fold difference in DDD can be observed between a low consumption group consisting of the Nordic countries, the Netherlands and the UK, versus a high consumption group that includes Korea, Greece, and the Slovak Republic (not reported in the table) (OECD 2015, p. 138).

6.3.2 Veterinary Consumption

Within the veterinary sector, it is possible to observe similar differences in the level of consumption of antimicrobials. In Table 6.2, two sets of data from a number of EU countries are presented. In the first column the total livestock biomass in the different countries is presented. This indicates the overall size of the livestock production in the country. In column two the antimicrobial consumption per kilogram biomass is presented for each country. It gives us the opportunity to compare levels of antimicrobial consumption in each country.

The major part of the antibiotic consumption in the veterinary sector is in the swine production (Eurostat 2014). In pig production, antimicrobials are widely used; for example, when young piglets - aged four to six weeks are separated from the sows. Changes in feed patterns often lead to diarrhea among the piglets, which is then treated with antimicrobials. As it can be seen in Table 6.2, we can observe similar major differences in the

Table 6.2 Consumption of antimicrobials by food-producing animals expressed as milligrams consumed per kilogram biomass in selected EU countries, 2012

	Total livestock biomass in 1000 tons	Milligrams antimicrobials per kilogram biomass
Sweden	783	13.5
Finland	511	23.8
Denmark	2.424	44.1
UK	6.749	66.3
France	7.618	99.1
Poland	3.908	132.2
EU mean (with population weight)	55.421	144.0
Portugal	996	157.1
Germany	8.338	204.8
Spain	6.996	242.0
Italy	4.500	341.0

Source: European Centre for Disease Prevention and Control et al. (2015, p. 29)

levels of antimicrobial use in the veterinary sector as we saw in the human sector. In Sweden, 13.5 milligrams of antimicrobials are used per kilo biomass, while the amount rises to 341 milligrams in Italy. Among the major meat producing countries, Denmark has the lowest level of antimicrobial use: 44.1 milligrams per kilo biomass, mainly used in swine production.

6.3.3 Patterns of AMR

If we look specifically at Europe and the EU, there is a trend toward both a North–South axis and an East–West axis in relation to consumption of antimicrobials. The Northern and Western European countries use fewer antimicrobials than the Southern and Eastern countries (European Centre for Disease Prevention and Control et al. 2015). This is the case both within the human and the veterinarian sector.

If we look more specifically at the relationship between antimicrobial consumption and AMR, it is well-known that a high level of antimicrobial consumption increases the AMR in different pathogens. It is well-documented that the overall level of AMR is lower in Denmark than in most other European countries (European Centre for Disease Prevention and Control 2015). This is the case for several different pathogens.

Table 6.3 *Klebsiella pneumoniae*

Percent	Country
0–1	Island
1–5	**Denmark**, Sweden, Norway, Finland, Holland, UK, Austria
5–10	Germany, Belgium, Ireland
10–25	France, Spain, Portugal, Estonia
25–50	Italy, Romania, Czech Republic, Latvia, Lithuanian
50–	Poland, Greece, Hungary, Slovakia

Percentage (%) of invasive isolates with combined resistance to fluoroquinolones, third-generation cephalosporins, and aminoglycosides in selected EU countries, 2014

Source: European Centre for Disease Prevention and Control (2015, p. 27, fig. 3.10)

Table 6.3 presents the level of AMR in a number of EU countries for one specific pathogen, *Klebsiella pneumonia*. *Klebsiella pneumonia* can cause a number of different infections, especially among humans with an already weakened immune system, and is especially prevalent in connection with urinary tract diseases.

Table 6.3 indicates the extent to which resistance to fluoroquinolones, third-generation cephalosporins, and aminoglycosides is found in *Klebsiella pneumonia* bacteria in the EU countries. Especially in the eastern and southern parts of the EU, there are high levels of multi-resistance bacteria. Similar low levels of AMR are found in the Nordic countries (and the UK, Holland, and Austria). The observed tendencies with regard to *Klebsiella pneumonia* can also be seen in connection with several other bacteria (ECDC 2015).

The spread of AMR in different regions of the EU correlates strongly with the amount of antimicrobials used in the different regions. Countries with low antimicrobial consumption—such as the Nordic countries—have low levels of AMR, while countries with high antimicrobial consumption—Italy for example—have high levels of AMR.

6.4 Governmental Structures in Denmark

Many years ago, the well-known German sociologist Max Weber famously distinguished between three types of social action, which he called instrumental, value-oriented, and traditional (Weber 1968). Instrumentally oriented social action refers to actions where people act in line with their interest. Value-oriented forms of social action refer to actions where people act in line with their values, while traditional forms of social actions reflect actions motivated by tradition.

When principals—such as governments—initiate regulatory initiatives in order to influence the behavior of the agents (the population or selected parts of the population), the initiatives often tend to be formed around the three above-mentioned types of social actions. Some governmental initiatives try to regulate citizens' behavior by developing incentive structures that appeal to the instrumental-oriented types of social action. Citizens are rewarded or punished if they behave in line with or in opposition to the stipulations set by the authorities. Other initiatives try to appeal to the citizen's values and stress the overall normative value of certain actions. Finally, efforts are made to change traditional forms of behavior by trying to establish new traditions and new forms of behavior.

In this section, we analyze some of the regulatory initiatives taken by Denmark authorities during the last 20 years in order to reduce consumption of antimicrobials. We make a distinction between initiatives that have tried to influence antimicrobial users' behavior with regard to the three above-mentioned types of social action (instrumental, value, and tradition). We also present cases from both the human and the veterinary sectors.

Within principal–agent theory, information is a central and crucial parameter in the relationship between the principal and the agent. As stated previously, one of the major problems that a principal has in order to govern an agent is lack of information about the area the principal is trying to regulate. It is the agent who has the information about how a given type of action is optimized in line with the interest of the principal. However, the agent could withhold information if it is not in the agent's interest to provide the principal with knowledge and information transparency. In the literature, it is therefore often observed that principals try to gather information independently of the agents whom they are governing.

This observation is confirmed in connection with the Danish government's efforts to reduce antimicrobial consumption and AMR. Over the last 20 years, the Danish state has developed a system of surveillance that measures antimicrobial consumption (and AMR) within both the human and veterinarian sectors. The system is based on registrations of prescriptions of antimicrobials by veterinarians and human doctors (from general practices, hospitals, etc.). Data from the surveillance system are published yearly in the DANMAP reports (DANMAP 2016). This surveillance system is a precondition for the Danish state acting as a principal in relation to users of antimicrobials. It provides information about patterns of user activity, enabling the state and public authorities to establish baselines and benchmark criteria for antimicrobial consumption. This is very much in line with the governmentality observations discussed in Chap. 1.

DANMAP—as the surveillance system is called—is probably one of the most reliable and detailed national systems that measures antimicrobial consumption in the world. It gives government agencies and health professionals important access to knowledge about which types of antimicrobials have been used and which types of diseases they have been applied to both in the veterinary and human areas.

We now present some examples of governmental initiatives taken by the Danish state and by the public authorities in order to reduce the overall consumption of antimicrobials. The examples show how Danish authorities use different types of means in the principal–agent relations depending on which types of users of antimicrobials are being targeted. The examples also reflect the three types of social action developed by Weber. Some of the examples are well-known as regulatory praxis in other countries, while others have been developed and used mainly in Denmark.

The first set of examples relates to some of the general information campaigns about antimicrobial consumption that have been launched by Danish public authorities. It is well-documented that especially general practitioners find themselves confronted with patients who can be very eager to obtain antimicrobials. In the health literature, this has been described as 'prescribing under pressure' (Stivers 2007) indicating that doctors are under pressure to prescribe antimicrobials beyond the medical need in order to fulfill the expectations and demands of their patients. In order to increase public awareness of the consequences of misuse of antimicrobials, various campaigns have been initiated (e.g. www.antibiotikaellerej.dk). These campaigns often target the population in general and focus on the overall consequences of a high consumption of antimicrobials. The risk that the use of antimicrobials will lead to the development of resistance is a core message in such campaigns. In that situation, the principal—the public authority—tries to use value-based types of arguments in order to change the behavior of the population. The principal appeals to the values of agents by stressing the risk of resistance development and its consequences for the general population.

The second type of governmental initiative is more directly oriented toward changing existing habits among selected groups in the health system. This has been developed under the heading 'antimicrobial stewardship' and is being used increasingly in Danish hospitals and other medical institutions. The use of antimicrobial stewardship is widespread in many other countries, for example, in the UK. Antimicrobial stewardship consists of various initiatives intended to increase awareness of how antimicrobials can be used most effectively. In this context, the focus is on how governmental authorities try to increase hygiene standards in hospitals and other facilities by changing the daily habits of the employees. Hygiene is an important factor in combating infections and the over-use of antimicrobials. Low levels of hygiene increase the spread of infections and drive up the need for use of antimicrobials. Simple measures such as washing hands have for many years been an important way to reduce the risk of spreading bacteria and infections at hospitals. However, in order to reduce the spread, even more, hospitals increasingly provide germicides to the health staff. Hands are routinely washed in germicides in order to reduce the spread of bacteria and need for antimicrobials.

In this context, the principal, here represented by the hospital management, tries to support the development of new habits among agents (health personal) by providing germicides that shall be used routinely by the staff. By implementing these new habits antibiotic consumption (and AMR) is expected to go down within the hospital sector.

Punishment and reward—instrumental rationality—also plays a central role in Danish governmental initiatives to reduce the overall consumption of antimicrobials. The principal tries to change the behavior of the agents through the use of punishment and rewards. Here, we will focus on Danish swine production, showing how various governmental initiatives have influenced the consumption of antimicrobials in the swine production sector.

Here, we will discuss two initiatives aimed at controlling antimicrobial consumption in swine production: the ban on the use of antimicrobials as growth promoters, introduced in Denmark from the mid-1990s through 2000 (and in the rest of EU in 2005), and the introduction of the so-called 'yellow card' (taken from soccer-football) in 2010, which regulates the amount of antimicrobials that a swine farmer can use in his or her production and stipulates a possible fine for over-use.

In Table 6.4, data for Danish antimicrobial consumption in the veterinarian sector are presented from 1994 to 2015. Consumption is measured in tons of active antimicrobial agents. The figures regarding the veterinary sector do not distinguish between the types of animals (swine, cattle, poultry, etc.) on which antimicrobials are used. In fact, the majority of Danish veterinary sector antimicrobial consumption takes place in swine production. Hence, changes in levels of consumption relate primarily to changes in consumption in swine production.

The figures show that the use of antimicrobials within the veterinary sector was at its highest in 1994. More than 200 tons of active agents were used in the sector. In 2015, antimicrobial consumption had fallen to around 110 tons of active agents.

Looking at the effects of the gradual introduction of the ban on the use of antimicrobials as growth promoters, it is clear from Table 6.4 that it had quite an impact on the overall consumption. In five years, overall consumption in the veterinary sector fell dramatically. In 1994, the overall consumption was 208 tons; in 1999 it had been reduced to 73 tons.

From 2000 onward, however, Table 6.4 shows an increase in the consumption, to 135 tons in 2009. This increase lies in the medical use of antimicrobials. The data indicate the difficulty in identifying when antimicrobials are being used as growth promoters and when they are used for medical reasons.

Looking at the development of the overall consumption of antimicrobials in the veterinary sector from 1994 to 2009 from a principal–agent perspective, one can say that the principal (the government) sought to reduce antimicrobial consumption due to the risk of AMR. In order to fulfill this goal, the government introduced a ban on antimicrobial use as growth promoters. Use of antimicrobials for medical reasons was still permitted without limitation. The agents (the swine producers and the

Table 6.4 Prescribed antimicrobial agents for animals, Denmark, different years, in tons

Year	Overall consumption in tons	Part of the overall consumption that is used as growth promoting antimicrobials, in tons
1994	208	118
1995	143	93
1996	153	105
1997	159	106
1998	109	51
1999	73	8
2000	80	0
2001	90	0
2002	96	0
2003	103	0
2004	114	0
2005	114	0
2006	116	0
2007	124	0
2008	121	0
2009	135	0
2010	132	0
2011	117	0
2012	119	0
2013	121	0
2014	119	0
2015	112	0

Source: Based on DANMAP (2016, p. 31, fig. 4.1)

veterinarians) reacted as expected by the principal and reduced their consumption. However, from 2000 onward, consumption increased again. This time, antimicrobials were not used as growth promoters but (ostensibly) as medicine.

The data show that it was difficult for the principal (the government) to continue to change the behavior of the agents (the swine producers). The principal had difficulties managing the distinction between antimicrobials used as growth promoters versus antimicrobials used for medical reasons. This can be seen as an example of asymmetrical access to information.

The yellow card, which is another second governmental initiative targeting swine producers, was introduced in 2010. The introduction of the yellow card can be seen as the principal's (the government's) response to the information asymmetry and to the undesired (by the principal) increase in antimicrobial use among swine producers from 2000 onward. Part of this increase in antimicrobial consumption in the swine production relates to increases in the overall production of swine. The number of produced swine increased in this period.

The yellow card initiative makes it possible to measure the exact amount of antimicrobials that each swine producer uses and for which type of medical purpose (diarrhea, urine-infections, etc.). Each swine producer's consumption of antimicrobials (per pig) is compared with the average consumption of antimicrobials in all swine herds in Denmark. The average consumption of antimicrobials per swine is used as a baseline for assessing the consumption level by a specific swine producer. If the consumption exceeds the average by a specific amount, the swine producer will receive a yellow card and will have to develop an action plan for reducing consumption. The yellow card initiative led to a decrease in the consumption of antimicrobials from 2010 and forward. According to the European Medicines Agency: 'The overall consumption of veterinary antimicrobial agents decreased 7% from 2010 to 2012, mainly due to new regulations directed towards the 5–10% of pig producers that used most of the antimicrobial agents' (European Medicines Agency 2014, p. 65).

The introduction of the yellow card system can be seen as a means by which the government, acting as the principal, handles the information asymmetry with regards to the agents (the swine producers). By developing baselines to compare consumption of antimicrobials among different swine producers, the principal becomes able to identify the specific swine producers who are not acting in accordance with the goal of the principal.

6.5 Conclusion

This chapter focused on the factors which caused overall consumption of antimicrobials to be lower in Denmark than in a number of other countries. This is the case for both the human and the veterinary sector.

In analyzing Danish governmental initiatives directed against reducing antimicrobial consumption in order to reduce the spread of AMR, we used a theoretical framework combining both a collective action perspective and principal–agent theory. It was shown that when the government acts as the principal, it uses different types of regulation depending on which type of agents it is targeting. In some situations, the initiatives are based on value-oriented types of social action. This is the case, for example, with regard to more general awareness-raising campaigns aimed at the public. In other situations, the government deployed more instrumentally oriented types of regulation. This was the case with regard to the swine producers and the government's attempt to reduce antimicrobial consumption in the pig production sector. It was shown that the information asymmetry between the principal (government) and the agents (the swine producers and the veterinarians) constituted a special challenge for the government.

References

Aarestrup, F. M. (1999). Association between the consumption of antimicrobial agents in animal husbandry and the occurrence of resistant bacteria among food animals. *International Journal of Antimicrobial Agents, 12*, 279–285.

Aulakh, P. S., & Gencturk, E. F. (2000). International principal–agent relationships: Control, governance and performance. *Industrial Marketing Management, 29*, 521–538.

DANMAP. (2016). DANMAP (2015)—Use of antimicrobial agents and occurrence of antimicrobial resistance in bacteria from food animals, food and humans in Denmark. Retrieved from http://www.danmap.org/Downloads/Reports.aspx

Elgie, R. (2002). The politics of the European Central Bank: Principal-agent theory and the democratic deficit. *Journal of European Public Policy, 9*, 186–200. https://doi.org/10.1080/13501760110120219

European Centre for Disease Prevention and Control. (2015). Antimicrobial resistance surveillance in Europe 2014. *Annual Report of the European Antimicrobial Resistance Surveillance Network* (EARS-Net), Stockholm.

European Centre for Disease Prevention and Control, European Food Safety Authority, European Medicines Agency. (2015). ECDC/EFSA/EMA first joint report on the integrated analysis of the consumption of antimicrobial agents and occurrence of antimicrobial resistance in bacteria from humans and food-producing animals: Joint Interagency Antimicrobial Consumption and Resistance Analysis (JIACRA). *Report of EFSA Journal, 13*, 4006. https://doi.org/10.2903/j.efsa.2015.4006

European Commission. (2015). ECDC/EFSA/EMA first joint report on the integrated analysis of the consumption of antimicrobial agents and occurrence of antimicrobial resistance in bacteria from humans and food-producing animals. *European Food Safety Authority*.

European Medicines Agency. (2014). *Sales of veterinary antimicrobial agents in 26 EU/EEA countries in 2012*. Fourth ESVAC report, London.

Eurostat. (2014). Pig farming in the European Union: Considerable variations from one Member State to another. *Statistics in Focus* 15/2014.

Gelband, H., Miller-Petrie, M., Pant, S., Gandra, S., Levinson, J., White, A., & Laxminarayan, R. (2015). *The state of the world's antibiotics 2015*. Washington, DC: The Center for Disease Dynamics, Economics & Policy.

OECD. (2015). *Health at a glance 2015: OECD indicator*. Paris: OECD Publishing.

Stivers, T. (2007). *Prescribing under pressure: Parent-physician conversations and antibiotics*. Oxford: Oxford University Press.

Weber, M. (1968). *Economy and society: An outline of interpretive sociology*. New York: Bedminster Press.

WHO. (2017). *Critically important antimicrobials for human medicine*, 5th revision. Geneva: WHO.

7

My Life as a Pig: MRSA and the Control of Life in Contemporary Pig Production

Lars Fynbo

7.1 Introduction

Rather than analysing action by deciphering its different 'layers', the actor–network theory (ANT) enables social science to study action in terms of 'versions' (Latour 2005, p. 244). The theory points out that within social networks, constantly formed by interrelated and interacting *actants*, action is always 'a version of action'. By constituting the time and space of the action, described somewhat similarly by Goffman (1967) as 'where the action is', an actor-network is at the same time enabling and enabled by the interactions of the actants constituting the network. We can thus understand an actor-network as constituted by interaction and as constituting action (Latour et al. 2012).

Where sociology has tended to conceive sociality more as 'typifications' of face-to face encounters (Berger and Luckman 1966, p. 43ff; Goffman 1967) or different layers of 'self' (Mead 1934; Wolfe 1991) and

L. Fynbo (✉)
VIVE – The Danish Center for Social Science Research,
Copenhagen, Denmark
e-mail: lafy@vive.dk

C. S. Jensen et al. (eds.), *Risking Antimicrobial Resistance*,
https://doi.org/10.1007/978-3-319-90656-0_7

as constituted by epistemological variations of knowledge and truth (Foucault 1970), ANT approaches the social focusing of how action is situated in a network (Latour 1993) or how a network is always in effect '*whenever action is to be redistributed*' (Latour 2011: 797, italics in original). According to Latour, different social realities are always socially constructed through changes or redistributions. Social construction always implies 'an *increase* in realism' (Latour 2005, p. 92) and social interaction is always a matter of situated action. Latour's conception of the 'social' is further used to 'deploy the associations that have rendered some state of affairs solid and durable' (Latour 2005, p. 93). In this chapter and in line with Latour, I thus conceive the social as a social construction which operates wherever and whenever multiple and relational interaction (Mol 1999, p. 75) becomes solid and durable.

As one of the 'most influential paradigms of nature-society relations' (Castree 2002, p. 115), one branch of contemporary ANT, called 'nature-society theory' (Royle and Loftus 2017), focuses on the agency of 'natural science objects', such as mushrooms (Tsing 2014), coffee (Mol 2012), and meerkats (Candea 2013). These studies relate to Marilyn Strathern's (2002) contemporary method, in which different fields of knowledge can be compared in terms of their perception. Hence, Tsing (2014) studies a fungal spore as an ethnographic *subject* by having the spore itself narrate a tale of life as a complex and unpredictable, sometimes disastrous, sometimes fortuitous process. Tsing's study, based as it is on the 'self-presentation' of a fungal spore, leads to somewhat 'intuitively structured' conceptions of 'other worlds' (ibid., p. 5) set up by 'continuous, indeterminately growing…interactive trajectories…without any central administration' (Rayner 1997, quoted in Tsing 2014, p. 11). Tsing's analysis thus opposes what she understands as a general tendency of modernity to control and administer nature.

Between December 2014 and 2015, I interviewed 30 pig farmers from two areas in Denmark and two veterinarian surgeons, as well as conducted field trips to 20 different pig farms. The sample of interviewees includes some of the largest pig producers in Denmark. The two animal surgeons whom I also interviewed were all specialized in contemporary production of pigs. The vets were associated with two large veterinary clinics, at the time of the interviews, covering more than 40 per cent of Denmark's entire pig production. Denmark, with less than six million people, is one of the world's major pig producers. In 2014, Danish farmers produced about 30 million pigs (Danish Agriculture & Food Council 2014), as well as eight million pigs dying during production (Ministry of Food, Agriculture and Fisheries of Denmark 2012). In this chapter, I focus on the control of pigs and the administration of microscopic life in contemporary pig farms based on the qualitative data generated from research with key actors within Danish pig farming.

7.2 Microbes and Antimicrobial Agents

To study modern-day pig production from a nature–science perspective we first need to look at how bacteria—according to scientific knowledge—behave in their natural environments and how they react to various stimuli, such as antibiotics. The modern understanding of antibiotics dates to 9 April 1880, when Scottish surgeon Alexander Ogston presented his studies of staph bacteria to the international scientific community in Berlin (Newsom 2008, p. 371; Ogston 1881). Ogston agreed with the findings of several contemporaries that infections were caused by 'micro-organisms' ('micrococci') being introduced into different types of animal or human life forms:

> When....injections were made with pus containing micrococci....the animals refused food, sat cowering in a retired place in their cage, were listless and apathetic, their coat was disordered and sometimes wet, their eyes were kept closed save when startled, and the mice showed purulent conjunctivitis and glueing together of the eyelids described by Koch in his experiments on septicæmia. (Ogston 1881)

However, Ogston also discovered large variations between different animals injected with the same type and number of pathogenic bacteria. Several test animals tended to fight off the micrococci-induced infections by themselves within about a week, and even the most virulent infections were ameliorated by fresh air. Ogston thus concluded that micrococci comprised a large family of pathogenic life forms causing numerous infectious diseases that were dependent on both their hosts and the surrounding climate.

In 1928, a year before Alexander Ogston passed away, another Scottish scientist revolutionized modern bacteriology and our conception of antimicrobial agency. Alexander Fleming's discovery of penicillin from 'ordinary nutrient broth' proved to be a milestone for the contemporary scientific conception of bacteria and antibiotics (Fleming 1929; Sykes 2001). Fleming (1929, p. 231f) tested different concentrations of penicillin on many different bacteria and found that penicillin had strong inhibitory effect on staphs and streptococci. Fleming (1929, p. 236) also noted that '[p]enicillin is non-toxic to animals in enormous doses'. The discovery of penicillin thus enabled solutions to bacterial infections that heretofore had not existed previously. Thus, in 1945, Fleming, together with Ernst B. Chain and Howard W. Florey, was awarded the Nobel Prize in Physiology or Medicine 'for the discovery of penicillin and its curative effect in various infectious diseases' (Nobel Media AB 2014).

According to the work of the modern medical pioneers, diseases are 'merely alterations of vital properties', that is, 'in the morbid form of life' (Foucault 1973, pp. 149, 154). From this perspective, bacteria are conceived as a natural pathological 'existence' with its own 'recognisable.... purpose' (Ogston 1881, p. 369), while antibiotics, similarly, are but a remedy that controls these pathological life forms. The administration of antimicrobial agents to bodies inhabited with bacteria thus becomes a matter of controlling one life form using another form of life.

7.3 Antibiotics and Modern-Day Farming

Whereas new machines, tools, and harvesting techniques played the major role in the industrial revolution of the late eighteenth and early nineteenth centuries, fertilizers and medicine have been central to the major increases in farm productivity since the mid-twentieth century (Brown 2010). Since the 1950s, antibiotics have thus been a key instrument for industrialized livestock farming all over the world (Boerlin and White 2013).

In Denmark, between 1990 and 2012, the total use of antimicrobial agents in animal farming more than doubled, from 53 to 116 tons active compound (The Danish Integrated Antimicrobial Resistance Monitoring and Research Programme (DANMAP) 2002, 2013). Recent diagnostics from DANMAP connect the heavy use of, especially, tetracycline with a current spread of methicillin-resistant staph bacteria, including the zoonotic clonal complex Methicillin-resistant Staphylococcus aureus (MRSA) CC398.

The fact that this clone of MRSA can spill over from animals to humans (as well as from humans to animals) (Kuehn 2012) has been an important factor in many of the most dangerous human epidemics and pandemics, such as bubonic plague, Marburg virus, AIDS and Ebola (Quammen 2012). Not surprisingly, MRSA CC398 has caused considerable public concern (see Chap. 8), being known among the Danish public as 'swine-MRSA'. The public concern has led to stronger demands for higher biosecurity standards at public hospitals, often including separating patients who have been tested positive for MRSA or who are suspected to be carriers of MRSA—such as pig farmers. There has also been a range of governance regulations aimed at pig farmers (see Chap. 6), varying from higher standards for biosecurity at the production sites to stricter surveillance of their use of antibiotics. The public conception of swine-MRSA also imposes a certain type of social stigma upon farmers, farmers' partners and children, and farmers' employees (see Chap. 8). There are occasional stories in the media about farmers' children having been critically confronted or bullied by peers (or peers' parents), sometimes excluded from birthday parties, sports events, and so on. Recently, a campaign led by an independent critic publicly warned the general population about having sex with people working within the pork industry.

7.4 A Pig's Life

In the middle of the sometimes-lively MRSA debate live the pigs, behind locked doors in secure environments closed off from the public. Before the age of 12 months, the pigs will have been transported to slaughterhouses to end their lives. During their short life on the pig farms, several somewhat minor objects and actions are important to the pigs at the different stages in their lives and for how the pigs may in fact become individual constructions of life.

To begin with, within the first couple of days of a pig's life, an average of two pigs die in each litter of eight to ten piglets. Depending on the farmers, the dead piglets are left together with the remains of the placenta for hours, even days, underneath the bars intended to keep the sow from squeezing her offspring. Even though different farmers set up different cages for the sows, some more ingeniously than others, they all fixate the sow to prevent her from squeezing her offspring. The somewhat macabre setup of a very big sow together with both her placenta, her living and her dead offspring, in a very small space is graphic evidence of the kind of control that humans exert over the pigs' lives. Within the first week of the pig's life, while the pigs are still together with the sow, a young farm worker, who in Denmark is often a woman of Eastern European origin and commonly referred to as a 'pig-girl', cuts away the male piglets' testicles with a special pair of tongs.

If possible, the castration occurs during his sleep, but the large number of castrations executed in the same space nevertheless leads to a great deal of shrieking among the many piglets. Castrations, argue the farmers, make the male pigs easier to handle because they become less territorial and aggressive. Castrations also improve the quality (and price) of the meat, supposedly removing an unpleasant taint from the meat. A week later, the same pig-girl uses a similar appliance to free all the piglets, male and female, of their tails, because, explain veterinary surgeons, 'tails are easy targets for other pigs' and thus 'likely to become infected'. To this day, even though tail cuttings on entire herds are in fact illegal in Denmark the practice is very common and tolerated by the visiting veterinary surgeons.

Alongside the internal and external bodily modifications, the piglets often begin a regime of three, five, or ten-day antibiotics treatments. Dietary doxycycline is added to their watering trough as a means of mass medicating an entire herd. Doxycycline belongs to the tetracycline family and is also used to treat certain bacterial diseases on humans such as chlamydia, pneumonia and syphilis. Farmers apply this type of broad-spectre antibiotic to entire herds of piglets in order to either cure an actual outbreak of diarrhoea or, in most cases, prophylactically so as to ensure that the young piglets do not develop an infection or get diarrhoea. This practice, which like the tail-cutting is a violation of existing rules, is also common. When asked about which type of antibiotics they would find it hardest to live without, several farmers cited doxycycline for its effectiveness in preventing outbreaks of diarrhoea amongst the piglets.

During this early stage of the pigs' lives, the following actants are important for the pigs: offspring mortality, fixation sow bars, pig-girls, testicles, tongs, castration, meat quality, tail docking, dietary doxycycline, mass medication, tetracycline, and diarrhoea.

When the piglets are about a month old, farmers separate them from their mothers and siblings, divide them by size and physical constitution (sick pigs are put together in a special 'sick bay') and move them into boxes in a new section called the 'climate sty'. According to farmers and vets, successful separations, that is separations that do not lead to outbreaks of diseases (mostly, diarrhoea), depend on the prior administration of doxycycline to the piglets. In the warmer and more humid climate sty, where the groups are of 20 to 30 small pigs, the pigs now have between three to five weeks to form the hierarchy in each herd while, at the same time, they must adjust from fluid to solid, protein-enriched food. During this transition and to prevent the pigs from getting diarrhoea, some farmers distribute a three-to-five-day antibiotics treatment with a tetracycline to entire herds. However, when the pigs are moved to the climate sties, most farmers tend to abort herd medication and from then on will then only treat individual pigs.

Based on my observations at this middle-stage of the pigs' lives, the following actants are active in constructing the pigs as objects: separation, climate sty, herd hierarchy, protein-enriched food, sick bay, and tetracycline. During this phase, the curious and playful young pigs often interact with the farmers through grunting and, when a recognizable farmer enters their bay, gnawing on the farmer's rubber boots. Similarly, some farmers get to know the personality of some of the pigs. For example, a weak and smallish pig can receive special treats, which are handfed so that the other, stronger pigs do not take them. Together with a small dose of antibiotics—to prevent post-delivery inflammations—one farmer served a Danish variant of cola to the sows each time they had given birth. If, however, the vet decides to put down and conduct an on-the-spot euthanasia, for instance, to see if the sick pick was carrying some type of organ disease, all the caring and special attention will cease immediately. Depending on the size of the pig farmers will put down a sick pig either by grabbing its hind legs and smashing its head to the concrete ground or by 'shooting' it in the head with a captive bolt gun. The heart continues drumming for several minutes after the pig has been cut open for the autopsy: another graphical evidence of the kind of control humans exert over the pigs' lives.

For the remaining three to four months of the pigs' lives, before the full-grown pigs are slaughtered, they live in a third type of stable, which is colder and less humid. In this stable, the pigs are again divided by size: first when moving from the climate sty and again when they have reached a certain weight and outgrown the stalls. During the last three to four months of the pigs' lives, farmers in Denmark are legally allowed to medicate only individual pigs; most often, due to a twisted joint causing inflammation or because of a sore bite or cut. However, at this stage of the pigs' lives, some farmers may also choose to utilize antibiotics for two other reasons (even though they breach the law). Firstly, farmers can maximize the growth of the pigs during their final stage prior to slaughter by feeding them or injecting them with one or more courses of tetracycline. 'When the slaughter pigs weigh about 70 kilos, and if you have some left-over medicine, you can boost their weight gain by adding medicine to their food', explained one of the veterinary surgeons somewhat bluntly. 'However', the vet emphasized, 'this is the sort of growth promotion that is no longer allowed'. A second reason farmers resort to antibiotics is to minimize the harm (and loss of growth) connected to large outbreaks of contagious disease or virus. The farmers can turn to antibiotics as a supplement even though the disease outbreak is not bacteriological. The logic behind this type of medication practice, which I observed at a couple of farms and was explained to me by both farmers and vets, is that 'medicine [i.e., antibiotics] helps boost the pigs back to normal; it gives them something to stand up with against the pressure of the virus'.

At the final stage of the pigs' lives, the terminus slaughter station becomes a more and more indispensable actant. The pigs, now living in relatively cold and dry environments, are not as prone to contracting internal bacteriological infections as they were earlier in their lives. Instead of bacteriological infections, farmers are now more concerned about how to fill up the transportation wagons to the slaughterhouse. Transportation fits in with the entire cycle of the whole production, so the wagons are scheduled to arrive on the same weekday all year round. Therefore, the pigs are kept by size to fit them into the transportation wagons as effectively as possible: 'empty space on the trucks is a waste of money, so the pigs must be ready and ready to go when the trucks arrive, which they do at eight o'clock every Monday all year around', explains one of the farmers whom I visited.

During this last stage of the pigs' lives, the time of the transportation to the slaughter station is the most significant actant for the pigs. Other actants are separation, inflammation and, for some farmers, illegal medication. As I will discuss in-depth in the last section of this chapter, some actants (like 'separation') remain active during the pigs' entire lifespan, whereas others are taken over by new significant actants (like 'sick bay' taken over 'diarrhoea').

7.5 Pigs and Antimicrobial Resistance

When asking farmers and veterinary surgeons about why they use antibiotics, their two most prominent responses were (1) in order to treat the sick pigs and (2) in order to ensure productivity and profit for their enterprises and families. During the entire process from birth to slaughterhouse transportation, farmers are concerned about the persistent risk of their herds catching contagious viral or antimicrobial diseases. 'There is always something lying in wait for your animals', explains a farmer, thereby underscoring the constant need for antibiotics.

Even though modern-day farming is strongly structured by the farmers earnings performancese and revenues, the administration of antibiotics—and the assessment of risks related to this type of farming—is not simply a problem to be solved by rational economic calculations. A 'sickness-concern', in other words, interacts with a 'profit-concern', contributing a certain social practice about the administration of the pigs' lives. This practice relies on the ready availability of medicine and the technical means of control that the farmers have developed over time, as well as scientific (and local, every day, and experience-based) knowledge about the nature of pigs and about bacteriological diseases and antimicrobial agents.

Currently, with the widely used application of antibiotics as a key tool for controlling the growth of the pigs throughout their brief lifespan, two relationships relevant to the connection between heavy use of antibiotics and antimicrobial resistance stand out as somewhat controversial for public health and for the lives of the pigs. Firstly, the dual functions of the veterinary surgeons (who are at the same time consultants and controllers) and their view of animal welfare in terms of cost-effectiveness. From a pig's perspective, this means that the pig can only be sick either if it does not gain weight (cost-effectively) or if it has been mistreated and has not had its welfare looked after. Within this relationship, sickness cannot be natural. Secondly, by assuming that pathogenic bacteria are not the norm, not something that the pigs carry 'naturally' or can live with, but rather an anomaly (see Chap. 8) to be eliminated via antibiotics, modern-day farmers and veterinary surgeons collaborate in forming a situation where 'the natural' is only something to be controlled and manipulated. They then produce nature through control, and by doing so, as a paradoxical consequence, risk not only the nature of the pigs but also, more broadly, public health and human nature.

In a Danish radio debate (DR 2014), Professor of Microbiology Hans Jørn Kolmos, an outspoken critic of the current high use of antibiotics in Danish farming, cited the risk of disrupting natural balances with medicine:

> Humans and animals live in a sort of natural balance with their microbiology. It's problematic to disturb this balance, for instance, with too much use of antibiotics. When we disturb our natural microbiology, we allow other microorganisms such as pathogenic bacteria to inhabit our organisms and cause infections.

Another outspoken critic of Danish farming's use of antibiotics, Professor at the National Food Institute in Denmark, Frank Møller Aarestrup, explains the prevalence of MRSA in pigs by focusing on the conditions under which pigs live:

> MRSA not only concerns the mere use of antibiotics. As a bacterial pathogen, it [MRSA] is not something that the pigs naturally carry as part of their nature. We must remember that in fact, these strains are not natural to the pigs. There are other reasons that it [MRSA] has become so prevalent in pigs.

According to these two scientific experts, the combination of a high use of antibiotics and fertile living conditions for pathogenic bacteria creates a risk of further proliferation of antibiotic-resistant bacteria such as MRSA. Aarestrup's solution to the problem, therefore, consists of a 'thorough sanitation', but, according to Aarestrup, this solution is 'not to be found, as if by magic, in a year or so'.

In the same debate, Kjeld Hansen, an independent critic of industrialized farming, further criticized the Danish veterinary surgeons' accommodation to what he called 'unnatural' industrialized farming:

> Since 2006, the administration of antibiotics has been controlled entirely by the animal surgeons, which is almost insane since the pigs don't by nature carry MRSA. It's unnatural. They get sick due to the way they are being treated as part of the production. It's the production of pigs that is sick, not the pigs themselves.

The survival and possible proliferation of MRSA, like that of any other bacterial life form, depends on its external conditions. Most importantly, MRSA needs a fertile habitat to survive and multiply, and it competes over this 'living space' with other bacteria as its natural enemies. The pathogen, like any other type of staph strain, appears to thrive in relatively stuffy buildings where many bodies live in very close proximity to each other: for example, modern hospitals and conventional pig farms. With their relatively dense mass of bodies, high use of antibiotics as well as many open wounds and/or infirm bodies, such facilities therefore offer pathogenic bacteria the most favourable of living conditions.

All the observed actants during my visits to the pig farms enforce more fertile habitats upon the pigs, either through applying antibiotics or by different types of separations. Blaser (2014) similarly describes how the overuse of antimicrobial agents affects the competition between non-pathogenic and pathogenic bacteria. Blaser points out how decades of overuse of antibiotics, particularly, on humans is steadily changing the existing bacterial constitutions of human beings. He argues that the bacteriological changes caused by decades of overuse of antibiotics create more fruitful conditions for pathogenic bacteria. Simply said, antibiotics intended to attack pathogenic bacteria also have an impact on useful and non-pathogenic bacteria; these derivative effects have adverse consequences and can end up improving the pathogens' living conditions. The positive effect of antibiotics on the pathogens is thus sometimes offset by its effect on other, non-pathogenic, bacteria.

7.6 Administering Nature on Danish Pig Farms

On one level, the actor-network that controls the lives of the pigs (in order to produce human food) consists of humans (farmers and veterinary surgeons) and of the scientific knowledge about microbes and antimicrobial agents. Hence, in accordance with Strathern's (2002) comparative method, the 'versions' of action that contribute agency to the pigs are the pig farmers and the veterinary surgeons and, more broadly, the scientific knowledge about pathogenic bacteria and antibiotics. Local knowledge and experience constitute a fourth version. When observing the different actants located in my study, we see that within this actor-network, different actants are active at different times of the pigs' lives. Table 7.1 shows the active actants in each of the three main stages of the pigs' lives.

The table shows how specific actants either transform into other, similar actants or become inactive. For example, the top row shows that initially, the farmers are not concerned about (offspring) mortality, viewing it as a normal part of pig production. Later, however, the farmers become more concerned about how to reduce pig mortality by separating the pigs more efficiently. This relationship between offspring mortality, common infections, sick bays, climate sty, and separations enables the farmers to conceive and manage the pigs as a mass of bodies rather than as individual

Table 7.1 Active actants in each of the three main stages of the pigs' lives

First stage	Second stage	Third stage
Offspring mortality	Separation from sow	Separation by size
Diarrhoea	Sick bay	Inflammation
Fixation sow bars	Climate sty	
Pig-girls	Herd hierarchy	
Tail docking		
Testicles		
Tongs		
Castration		
Dietary doxycycline	Tetracycline	Illegal medication
Tetracycline		
Mass medication		
Meat quality	Protein-enriched food	Slaughtering

animals. The next relationship aims at controlling the nature of the pigs' herd hierarchy by having the 'pig-girls' castrate the male pigs and cut the tales of all piglets while they are still small.

Medicine comprises the third relationship of the table. This relationship is fundamentally bound to the role of the veterinary surgeon and their role as the only one who can prescribe medicine for the farmers to use. However, all the farmers whom I interviewed had earned a certificate allowing them to distribute several antibiotics without first conferring with their animal surgeon. In fact, only herd medication depends on the professional assessment of an animal surgeon. This means that most of the medicine that the farmers distribute to the pigs is part of the daily routines on the farm rather than any kind of special measure. Firstly, at the beginning of the pigs' lives, the medical treatment supports the development of the piglets so that the farmers can separate them as early as possible from the sows without causing (too much) diarrhoea. Secondly, medications allow the farmers to perform the tail dockings, thereby, ensuring that the pigs do not catch tail infections when sorting out the herd hierarchies throughout their lives. Thirdly, medicine cures many diseases; some of them are somewhat expected (like diarrhoea), while others are more complicated and sometimes related to non-bacteriological diseases. In such circumstances, medicine is vital for modern-day pig farming. Furthermore, during the final stage of the pigs' lives, farmers can use medicine illegally to add a last-minute weight gain to the pigs before they are transported to the slaughterhouse. During my visits to the farms, I did not observe this kind of illegal administration of medicine first hand.

The transportation of the pigs, now conceived even more as a mass of bodies than at the beginning at their lives, becomes the last actant of the fourth relationship. This fourth relationship also comprises meat quality and protein-enriched food. Taken together, these actants enable the pigs to become a mere object of productivity that, throughout their lives, are destined to slaughter.

References

Berger, P. L., & Luckmann, T. (1966). *The social construction of reality*. New York: Anchor Books Publishing.

Blaser, M. J. (2014). *Missing microbes: How the overuse of antibiotics is fueling our modern plagues*. New York: Henry Holt & Company.

Boerlin, P., & White, D. G. (2013). Antimicrobial resistance and its epidemiology. In S. Giguère, J. F. Prescott, & P. M. Dowling (Eds.), *Antimicrobial therapy in veterinary medicine* (5th ed., pp. 21–40). Hoboken, NJ: John Wiley & Sons, Inc.

Brown, K. (2010). *Healing the herds: Disease, livestock economies, and the globalization of veterinary medicine*. Athens: Ohio University Press.

Candea, M. (2013). Habituating meerkats and redescribing animal behaviour science. *Theory, Culture & Society, 30*(7–8), 105–128.

Castree, N. (2002). False antitheses? Marxism, nature and actor-networks. *Antipode, 34*(1), 111–146.

Danish Agriculture & Food Council. (2014). *Statistics 2013: Pigmeat*. Report, Landbrug & Fødevarer, Copenhagen, June.

DANMAP. (2002). *Use of antimicrobial agents and occurrence of antimicrobial resistance in bacteria from food animals, foods and humans in Denmark*. ISSN 1600-2032.

DANMAP. (2013). *Use of antimicrobial agents and occurrence of antimicrobial resistance in bacteria from food animals, food and humans in Denmark*. ISSN 1600-2032.

Danmarks Radio. (2014). Radio programme. *Apropos: Resistens [Resistance]*. Danish Broadcasting Corporation, 24 February 2014.

Fleming, A. (1929). On the antibacterial action of cultures of a penicillium, with special reference to their use in the isolation of *B. influenzae*. *British Journal of Experimental Pathology, 10*, 226–236.

Foucault, M. (1970). *The order of things: An archaeology of the human sciences*. London: Tavistock Publications Limited.

Foucault, M. (1973). *The birth of the clinic: An archaeology of medical perception*. London: Tavistock Publications Limited.

Goffman, E. (1967). *Interaction ritual: Essays on face-to-face behavior*. New York: Anchor Books.

Kuehn, B. (2012). MRSA may move from livestock to humans. *The Journal of the American Medical Association, 308*(17), 1726.

Latour, B. (1993). *We have never been modern*. Cambridge, MA: Harvard University Press.

Latour, B. (2005). *Reassembling the social: An introduction to actor-network-theory*. Oxford: Oxford University Press.

Latour, B. (2011). Networks, societies, spheres: Reflections of an actor-network theorist. *International Journal of Communication, 5*, 796–810.

Latour, B., Jensen, P., Venturini, T., Grauwin, S., & Boullier, D. (2012). 'The whole is always smaller than its parts'—A digital test of Gabriel Tarde's monads. *The British Journal of Sociology, 63*(4), 590–615.

Mead, G. H. (1934). *Mind, self, & society from the standpoint of a social behaviorist*. Chicago: University of Chicago Press.

Ministry of Food, Agriculture and Fisheries of Denmark. (2012). *Avl af svin* [Pig farming]. Report, Copenhagen, January.

Mol, A. M. (1999). Ontological politics: A word and some questions. *The Sociological Review, 47*(S1), 74–89.

Mol, A. M. (2012). Layers or versions? Human bodies and the love of bitterness. In B. S. Turner (Ed.), *Routledge handbook of body studies* (pp. 119–129). London: Routledge.

Newsom, S. W. B. (2008). Ogston's coccus. *Journal of Hospital Infection, 70*, 369–372.

Nobel Media AB. (2014). The Nobel Prize in Physiology or Medicine 1945. Retrieved September 2016, from http://nobelprize.org

Ogston, A. (1881, March). Report upon micro-organisms in surgical diseases. *The British Medical Journal, 12*, 369–375.

Quammen, D. (2012). *Spillover: Animal infections and the next human pandemic*. New York: W. W. Norton & Company.

Royle, C. E., & Loftus, A. J. (2017). *Nature-society theory*. Oxford: Oxford Bibliographies.

Strathern, M. (2002). Foreword: Not giving the game away. In A. Gingrich & R. G. Fox (Eds.), *Anthropology, by comparison* (pp. xiii–xvii). London: Routledge.

Sykes, R. (2001). Penicillin: From discovery to product. *Bulletin of the World Health Organization, 79*(8), 778–779.
Tsing, A. L. (2014). Strathern beyond the human: Testimony of a spore. *Theory, Culture & Society, 31*(2–3), 221–241.
Wolfe, A. (1991). Mind, self, society, and computer: Artificial intelligence and the sociology of mind. *American Journal of Sociology, 96*(5), 1073–1096.

8

Social Stigmatization of Pig Farmers: Medical Perspectives on Modern Pig Farming

Carsten Strøby Jensen and Lars Fynbo

8.1 Introduction

In Denmark, the growing concern over the public health risks associated with the spread of resistant bacteria via conventional pig farming has caused some pig farmers and farm workers to experience social stigmatization. The stigmatization is rooted in the public's conception of antimicrobial resistance (AMR) as a significant threat to public health and by the publicity surrounding the presence of zoonotic bacteria such as methicillin-resistant *Staphylococcus aureus* (MRSA) in the majority of the Danish pig farms. According to the public conception, pig farming amplifies the risk of spreading AMR, and in addition, pig farmers and their family members may be infected with MRSA, and thus pose a risk to others.

C. S. Jensen (✉)
Department of Sociology, University of Copenhagen, Copenhagen, Denmark
e-mail: csj@soc.ku.dk

L. Fynbo
VIVE – The Danish Center for Social Science Research,
Copenhagen, Denmark
e-mail: lafy@vive.dk

C. S. Jensen et al. (eds.), *Risking Antimicrobial Resistance*,
https://doi.org/10.1007/978-3-319-90656-0_8

From a public health perspective, a zoonosis like MRSA clonal complex 398 (MRSA CC398) has attracted considerable attention. In the Danish public debate, MRSA CC398 is often referred to as 'swine-MRSA'. In this chapter, we therefore focus on two consequences of the conception of pig farming as a threat to public health: first, a renewed scientific concern over contemporary pig farming and second, the stigmatization of pig farmers both as a social group and as individuals.

From Britain's first known outbreak of 'flesh eating killer bugs' in 1994 and onwards (Brown 1994; Cartwright et al. 1995; Dixon 1996), health professionals, bacteriologists, and public health researchers, as well as the World Health Organization (WHO), have voiced growing concern over the continuous propagation of antibiotic-resistant bacteria in animals and its spread to human hosts. The emergences of new antibiotic-resistant strains constantly endanger, especially, hospitals' treatment of diseases that have been relatively easy to treat for more than half a century. Suddenly, these treatments do not work.

Among humans, the Danish health services in 2007 recorded 14 cases of MRSA CC398 infections among hospital patients. By 2014, the number of cases had increased to 1224 cases (DANMAP 2016). Along with the sharp increase in the number of reported cases of human MRSA infections, the proportion of MRSA CC398 among the total MRSA cases also increased. In 2007, MRSA CC398 comprised only 2.1% of all reported MRSA infections in Denmark, while this increased to 30.7% in 2013 (Statens Serum Institut 2014).

According to Voss et al. (2005) and van Cleef et al. (2010), modern farming contributes to the growth of antibiotic resistance. In Denmark, around 80 per cent of all conventional pig farms are infected with MRSA (Statens Serum Institut 2014). The prevalence of MRSA is high in rural areas with a high density of pig farms and almost absent in the large urban areas. Following statistics from Statens Serum Institut (2014) of the number of reported MRSA CC398 cases per 100,000 citizens in different geographical areas in Denmark we can almost draw a line between Greater Copenhagen (zero incidents per 100,000 citizens) and the rest of Zealand (zero to three incidents) in the urbanized eastern part of the country and Funen (12 incidents) and Jutland (11–30 incidents) in the more rural west. Köck et al. (2013) show similar results from the

Netherlands and Germany, thus, documenting how human infections are more prevalent in those areas with many pig farms.

In the same vein, several studies conclude that pig farmers are responsible for the spread of resistant bacteria to others and that pig farmers have a significantly high risk of catching MRSA CC398 from infected pigs (for example, Cox and Popken 2014). Relatives of pig farmers and farm workers are also at risk of catching the bacteria either through occasional visits to the pigsties or from infection transmitted by their partners or parents (Deiters et al. 2015). However, recent calculations from the Danish National Board of Health (2016) suggest that people who contract MRSA CC398 but who do not have daily or near-daily contact with infested pigs spontaneously 'drop' the bacteria within one to two weeks.

8.2 Contemporary Trends in Danish Pig Production and in the Production and Use of Antibiotics

Production of pigs for slaughter is a major industry in Denmark. In absolute numbers, Denmark occupies a 13th place among the world's pig producing countries, measured in kilograms of pork produced (Danish Agriculture & Food Council 2015, p. 10). Denmark produces approximately 30 million pigs annually, of which around 20 million are pigs for fattening and slaughter and 10 million are piglets (mostly, for export). In 2014, there were around 3500 farms with pigs, most of them with at least one employee. In Denmark, as in other agricultural countries, the use of antibiotics is an important component of pig production. The antibiotics are deployed mainly to fight bacterial diseases (typically diarrhea and pig cough), but antibiotics also have a positive effect on the rate at which the animals gain weight: the more antibiotics, the faster the growth. In the European Union (EU) and in Denmark, antibiotics have been banned as a growth promoter since 2005 (which is not the case, for example, in the USA).

The use of antibiotics in livestock production is strictly regulated through the so-called 'Yellow Card' scheme that monitors antibiotic consumption by individual farms on a monthly basis. The 'Yellow Card' scheme limits the amount of antibiotics that may be used per pig in a given herd, taking into account the size and age of the pig. The scheme is organized around a detailed registration of types and amounts of antibiotics used in a given situation. Antibiotic use is registered by the farmer and the veterinarian, who are also obliged to record for which disease antibiotics were used (e.g. diarrhea, joint inflammation, pig cough, etc.). Under law, antibiotics must be prescribed by a veterinarian. Unlike the situation in a number of other countries, veterinarians in Denmark may not profit on the sale of antibiotics themselves. The sale is organized through a third party such as a pharmacy or equivalent.

The regulations governing the use of antibiotics in pig production (and in other parts of livestock production) are intended to limit or reduce the use of antibiotics so as to prevent the risk of resistance development.

Table 8.1 gives an overview of the consumption of antibiotics in Danish pig production in 2014 by age group and type of antibiotics used.

Of the total consumption of antibiotics in Danish livestock production in 2014, pig production accounted for 76% (active substance share). The remainder was used in cattle, mink, chickens and hens (DANMAP 2015,

Table 8.1 Use of antimicrobial—pigs (kg active compound), different antimicrobial agents, age group, 2014, Denmark

Therateupic group	Sows and piglets	Weaners	Finishers	Total
Amphenicols	206	32	7	244
Aminoglycosides	1826	2446	222	4494
Cephalosporins	2	2	0	4
Fluoroquinolones	4	0	0	4
Other quinolones	0	0	0	0
Lincosamldes	480	729	858	2067
Macrolides	652	6899	3499	11,049
Pleuromutilins	602	3123	4395	8120
Penicillins, betalactamase sensitive	8883	1735	6056	16,675
Penicillins, others	3529	3259	1005	7784
Sulfonamides and trimethoprim	5631	2149	294	8074
Tetracyclines	2239	15,207	9403	26,850
Others	86	559	10	13,048
Total	24,140	36,131	25,749	86,020

Source: DANMAP (2015, p. 30)

p. 31). Total consumption of antibiotics in pig production was 86 tons of active substance in 2014. By comparison, around 60 tons of active substance was prescribed in the entire human area in 2014 (DANMAP 2015, p. 29, Table 4.1).

Among the types of antibiotics used in pig production, the consumption of tetracyclines is high (26,850 kg active compound). The extensive use of tetracyclines is believed to be one of the main factors causing development of MRSA. At the same time, in the broader context of resistance development, the consumption of cephalosporins and fluoroquinolones is very low. A special agreement was concluded within Danish agriculture to try to avoid using these types of antibiotics as they were viewed as being among the so-called 'critical antibiotics'. 'Critical antibiotics' are those that can be used when other groups of antibiotics have developed resistance. The fear was that increased consumption of these types of drugs, in pig production for example, would lead to resistance development even to these 'critical antibiotics'. In a number of other countries in the EU, the use of these critical antibiotics is also common in pig production, despite the risks mentioned (see also Chap. 6). It should also be noted that there is a relatively large consumption of macrolides in Denmark, although in the opinion of a number of European expert committees, the use of these types of antibiotics should be avoided in order to prevent resistance development.

Consumption of antimicrobials within pig production in Denmark is relatively low when compared with consumption in other countries in corresponding pig farms (see Chap. 6). However, it should also be noted that the overall amount of consumption of antimicrobials within the pig producing sector represents around 50% of the overall consumption of antimicrobials in Denmark (both within the human and the veterinarian sector).

8.3 Stigmatization

From a sociological point of view, stigmatization can be described as a process that 'reduces' a person 'possessing an attribute that makes him different from others' from 'whole and usual' to 'tainted' and 'discounted'

(Goffman 1963, p. 3). Stigmatization is a process that transforms a 'deviated' individual's 'social identity' from 'actual' to 'virtual'. Although stigma relates to different types of individual characteristics (for example, immoral behaviour or deformities), their effects on the stigmatized individual are the same: they experience that they deviate from the 'normal' (Goffman 1963, p. 5; Farigaiga 2009).

It is not the actual deviant attributes that make individuals who are stigmatized feel 'labelled', 'alienated', 'abolished', or 'not accepted'. Rather, it is the social element of the process of stigmatization (Link and Phelan 2001; Link 1987).

With a point of departure in Goffman's conception of stigma as inferring a potential discrepancy between the 'selves' of stigmatized individuals, newer research outlines three types of stigmatization processes: internalized stigmatization, socialized stigmatization, and institutionalized stigmatization (Corrigan et al. 2005; Herek et al. 2009; Livingston and Boyd 2010).

Internalized stigmatization refers to Goffman's original concept of 'actual self', whereby the stigmatized person acknowledges her or his deviance as natural and real. Socialized stigmatization refers to stigmatized persons identifying with a social group and with the stigmatization put on the entire group by other groups or social institutions. In relation to Goffman's terminology, this type of stigmatization process refers to the concept of 'virtual self' because the stigmatized persons likely do not accept their ascribed (virtual) deviant identity. Finally, institutionalized stigmatization occurs when institutions, for example hospitals, treat specific individuals or groups of people differently from the rest of the population because they are potentially dangerous.

8.4 Methods and Data

Overall, pig farmers are cautious about talking about their pig farming for fear of being subjected to criticism. We therefore decided to follow two different sampling strategies for the interviews with farmers and farm workers. Firstly, author two convinced an animal surgeon working with conventional pig farmers to take him on as an assistant for a week. During this week, he visited 14 different pig farms. The veterinarian introduced author two to each of the farmers and farm workers, and this enabled author two to briefly describe the research project, including our intention of generating data together with contemporary farmers and farm workers. Secondly, author two approached the head of a local farmers' organization who was involved in public debates about the actual risks related to AMR. After author two had attended a couple of public meetings in the local farming community, presenting himself, the research project, as well as our code of ethics (ASA 1999), this farmer agreed to an interview as well as allowing us to interview some of his employees. Further, we used snowball sampling (Biernacki and Waldorf 1981). After three rounds of snowballing, we ended the data generation process. All in all, 30 farmers and farm workers were interviewed, and our initial, descriptive analysis showed that data began saturating.

Simultaneously with the qualitative interviews with the pig farmers, author one selected and interviewed 21 stakeholders and experts within the public health and veterinary sectors. These interviews allowed the experts and stakeholders to relate their individual perception of AMR as a public health risk. When interviewing the experts, author one used two strategies: firstly, he interviewed a number of scientific experts within the field of antibiotic consumption, for example, microbiologists. Secondly, he interviewed members of several organized interests groups representing, for example, human medical doctors and veterinarians.

As the data in this chapter is based primarily on qualitative interviews, it should be noted that we cannot say to what extent the observations are representative for all medical experts, stakeholders, and pig farmers. We would need to use survey methods in order to evaluate the representativeness of our interviews.

8.5 AMR from a Public Health Perspective

A number of the expert and stakeholder interviews voiced general concerns over the fact that veterinary surgeons prescribe medicine intended for use by humans to farm animals in large quantities. The interviewees also criticized the kind of production that now comprises contemporary pig farming and questioned the willingness of farmers and farm workers to acknowledge the risk of AMR related to this type of agriculture. One of the interviewed (human) medical doctors forecast future potential problems with AMR related to pig farming:

> And the problem is … that if you get sick and if you have these resistant bacteria, then you cannot be treated. Then you will die of pneumonia because it might not be treatable. And this will also apply to the farmer and his two-year-old son if they become sick from the bacteria. Then we cannot treat them [in the future].

This interviewee viewed contemporary pig farming as causing the threat of resistant bacteria and cited pig farmers' lack of willingness to acknowledge the threats emanating from AMR. Pig farmers were often described as being irresponsible and thus normatively deviant because of the fatal consequences that their risky—and immoral—behaviour would presumably have for the general population.

Another interviewee, a microbiologist at a large regional hospital, also criticized the farmers because of what he considered their excessive use of antimicrobials in pig production.

> So please stop using so much tetracycline or reduce the use as much as possible. Try to do what we suggest: Identify the one pig that is sick; isolate it and then treat just this one pig. Do not treat the whole herd of pigs. And don't have so many pigs together in one small enclosure

This interviewee thus criticized the pig farmers for putting their business considerations ahead of animal welfare and the general health of the population. According to him, farmers have too many pigs living together in small enclosures, which increases the risk of spread of bacterial diseases. And these diseases then have to be treated using antimicrobials such as tetracycline. Similarly, pig farmers (and the veterinarians) use herd medication in order to decrease the workload related to treating sick pigs. The use of antimicrobials in herds instead of being administered to individual animals dramatically increases the risk of AMR.

Another interviewee argued that overuse of antimicrobials and the possible increase in AMR is closely related to modern pig production. For example, piglets are taken away from the sows very early in order to make them grow faster. This increases the likelihood that they get diarrhoea. The interviewee states:

> Access to antimicrobials established a certain type of pig farming, which is bad both for nature and the environment. It is a kind of system failure that so much antimicrobials are used in pig production. This is mainly because piglets are taken away from the sows too early in order to make them grow more. They are given solid food at a time when their digestive system cannot handle it. And so the piglets get diarrhea and need to be treated with antimicrobials. [...] In this respect, it is correct when the pig farmers argue that they only treat sick animals; however, *all* the pigs get sick [due to forms of production]

The interviewee here argues that pig farmers might be correct when they say that they only treat sick pigs with antimicrobials. However, the sick pigs are largely a foreseeable result of the forms of production. Modern pig production is dependent on farmers' use of antibiotics and other types of antimicrobials. In this sense, the pig farmers and the agricultural sector have a huge responsibility for the general development of AMR not only among their pig herds, but in Danish society generally.

In another interview, a medical doctor stressed how the use of antimicrobials among pig farmers influences their environment more directly. This is especially visible in connection with the spread of MRSA. It is mostly the pig farmers themselves who risk becoming carriers of resistant bacteria. However, when they and their families move around in their local community, the resistant bacteria can spread to other humans who are not directly in contact with pigs.

The doctor warns: 'Now they [the MRSA infections] pop up. They have spread from the pig farms. First they are carried by the farmers; then his daughter gets it. Then she goes to school and spreads it further around'.

8.6 Experienced Stigmatization among Pig Farmers

> When I go to a veterinarian congress abroad, I am usually very popular. Questions like: 'How can you manage to produce pigs so efficiently in Denmark' [and with such a low level of use of antimicrobials], are very common; They [the veterinarian colleagues] cannot understand how we do it ... When I am at home in Denmark, it is totally different. Here it is more like we are compared with rapists; it's very strange. But I have learned to

> live with it. It's like some persons drinking café latte in cafes in Copenhagen have decided that they don't like the agricultural forms of production. They don't like the kind of pig production we have in Denmark. It's very strange, especially when we compare it to how pig production is managed in other countries. You know, we are far far ahead in Denmark.

These remarks come from one of the veterinarians we interviewed in connection with our research. To a large extent, they represent the feelings expressed by many of the interviewed pig farmers and their families. They feel looked down upon and that they are being scolded; and they feel that they are encountering unfair accusations. They feel that they are unfairly treated, and even stigmatized.

According to Goffman's (1963) theory, an internalized stigma results from the merging of a person's 'virtual' and 'actual' selves. Internalized stigmatization, in other words, refers to the process during which a stigmatized person learns to acknowledge her- or himself according to the image (the virtual self) presented by the stigmatizers.

In real life situations internalized stigmatization is always a matter of nuance. The issue is how much does a stigmatized person connect their actual self-conception to the virtual self presented by the stigmatizers? In our sample, the internalized stigmatization process shows wide variations. Some farmers are more sympathetic towards accepting themselves and their use of antibiotics as entailing a risk to society, while others strongly resist any attempts at such a reduction of virtual to actual selves; they refuse to conceive themselves as morally irresponsible risk-bearers.

It is especially the more senior farmers, who may be partly retired but still remain very active in the daily life on the farms, who tend to either completely dismiss the criticism from the outside world, for example, as 'pure gibberish', 'fabrications from a few madcaps who have nothing better to do than befoul our farming', and so on, or who play down the risk associated with pig farming in Denmark by comparing it with the risk presented by 'foreign farm workers carrying MRSA across the borders', the 'feeding of antibiotics to pigs in China, Spain […] and Poland' as well as highlighting the 'absence of [antibiotic] regulations in Southern Europe'. One senior farmer points towards possible disease carriers outside of the stables:

> I've been thinking that, yes, some farms may have MRSA, but what about the forest animals? If we go down to the creek and into the forest, who knows what we may catch from the animals there? When the diseases travel overland, don't you think that maybe the forest animals and not the pigs are responsible?

All the senior farmers whom we interviewed had produced pigs for two, three or four decades. They have experiences from the era before AMR became a known threat and when farmers' use of antibiotics was completely without regulation. Without doubt, the senior farmers have had to incorporate great changes in both their production routines and in their perception of risk related to their production, especially over the last ten years. With their particular experience, the senior farmers tended to be more accustomed to disputing with critics and, thus, responding more categorically to the present criticism related to AMR.

Where the senior farmers are largely immune to criticism, their younger family members or younger colleagues are more affected by different types of public criticism. A young farmer explains that the criticism affects him differently depending on whether he sees himself as a 'farmer' or a 'person':

> And I sincerely believe that the media is more concerned about people's desire for a good story than about telling the truth. Our use of antibiotics is far below our threshold. Over the last five years, we've not once exceeded 50 per cent of our maximal allowance of antibiotics. Not once. So am I really that bad, you know? As bad as the esteemed professors say that I am? I don't think so.

The young interviewees, it seems, accept the major premise that excessive use of antibiotics in pig production entails a real risk. However, contrary to the generalized image of pig farmers as a uniform group, they also see themselves as individual farmers capable of producing pigs responsibly. They therefore repudiate merging their actual self (as responsible individuals) with the attributed virtual self of the concerned public health experts.

Two other younger interviewees feel more embarrassed than the interviewees mentioned above, being more affected by the public conception of pig farmers as dangerous. One of them, who was the only interviewee that had been tested positive for MRSA CC398, explains how he often tries to 'pass' (Goffman 1963) as a non-farmer rather than admitting that he produces pigs:

> I try to stay a little ahead of things by downplaying my involvement in conventional farming. You saw how I treat the pigs, right? And they are not mistreated, right? But, of course, they get sick. Right now, we have a lot of problems with the flu, like I told you, the H1N1 virus, right? So right now our medicine balance is in the red, and we have to keep a really tight rein on what we do. But when I talk to people who are not farmers, I'd never talk about any of this. No way. I have to think about how they'll approach my kids and my family, so I don't normally mention that I'm a farmer or that I have MRSA.

8.7 Conclusion: Risk, Uncertainty, and Stigmatization

The relationship between public health concerns and pig farming, which results in the stigmatization of the pig farmers, rests on two different approaches to the risk of AMR and especially the risk of zoonotic MRSA CC398. First, public health is rational and conceives the risk of MRSA rationally, thereby arguing that, since pig farming is associated with the risk and spread of pathogenic bacteria, pig farmers are in all probability contagious. In the secondary health sector, this rational perception of pig farmers causes hospitals to incorporate special procedures for pig farmers and their families, such as private wards, thereby reducing the danger of infection to other patients.

Secondly, contemporary risks are based on uncertainty (see Chap. 1). That is, the conception of risk is based on the perception of uncertainty. Therefore, even though most people will agree that antimicrobial resistant zoonotic pathogens should give rise to concern, the actual risk of, for example, MRSA CC398 is still not clear. In Denmark, the actual harm caused by MRSA CC398 so far have been minor, certainly nowhere near the measured cases of other documented epidemics and pandemics.

According to our analysis, it is the different understanding of the relation between risk and uncertainty between the public health officials and the farmers that leads to the stigmatization of the farmers as irresponsible, and it is the relationship between risk and uncertainty that causes stigmatization.

Our study shows that the relationship between public health and pig farming entails stigmatization of pig farmers and farm workers on two levels: on the individual level, pig farmers and farm workers sense a public hostility towards them as individual farmers. Hospitals put them in separate wards; their children may not be invited to birthday parties; they may simply hide the fact that they are pig farmers in order to avoid an awkward social situation. On the social level, a similar hostility aims at the farmers as a uniform social group: they are seen as irresponsible economic actors whose occupation may cause illness among an innocent public. The farmers and farm workers that we have interviewed for this study react differently to these individual and social stigmatization processes. Interviewees belonging to a senior generation of farmers are mostly seemingly unimpressed by the public's condemnation of pig farming as harmful and pig farmers as ignorant. On the contrary, the senior farmers often question the experts' knowledge, pointing towards nature and the human health sector as more serious risks to public health, and to contemporary farming. The senior farmers find the accusations aimed at their farming to be insulting. As such, their social stigmatization becomes an individual matter that they simply do not accept. The younger interviewees react differently to the stigmatization process than their senior colleagues. At the social level, the younger farmers admit that MRSA and other antimicrobial resistant pathogens can pose a risk to themselves, their families and to the general population. However, the young farmers do not see contemporary pig farming as chaotic or fundamentally dependent on medicine. All our interviewees felt that they—as well as all other farmers—need to control their need for antimicrobial agents, but they insist that as responsible farmers, they are already doing this. Furthermore, they argue that farmers are able to further refine their standards for biosecurity and that this will help reduce the veterinary demand for antimicrobial agents in the future. At the individual level, the younger farmers also react differently to the stigmatization process than the older generation. Where the senior farmers were indifferent or outrightly rejected the public health experts' conceptions of modern farming as irresponsible, the younger generations are clearly emotionally affected by the negative public image of contemporary farming. They fear for their children, who risk social exclusion, and when interacting with other people outside their local farming communities, to the extent that the young farmers often try to protect themselves by passing as non-farmers.

Besides showing that pig farmers tend to be stigmatized in connection with their use of antimicrobials, this article also shows that there are big differences in views on AMR within the human medical sector and the veterinarian/agricultural sector. The two sectors often blame each other for being responsible for the increasing problems with AMR in the overall society.

References

ASA—American Sociological Association. (1999). *Code of ethics and policies and procedures of the ASA committee on professional ethics*. Washington, DC: American Sociological Association.

Biernacki, P., & Waldorf, D. (1981). Snowball sampling: Problems and techniques of chain referral sampling. *Sociological Methods & Research, 10*(2), 141–163.

Brown, N. (1994). Dawn of the post-antibiotic age? *British Medical Journal, 309*, 615.

Cartwright, K., Logan, M., McNulty, C., et al. (1995). A cluster of cases of streptococcal necrotizing fasciitis in Gloucestershire. *Epidemiology & Infection, 115*(3), 387–397.

Corrigan, P. W., Kerr, A., & Knudsen, L. (2005). The stigma of mental illness: Explanatory models and methods for change. *Applied & Preventive Psychology, 11*, 179–190.

Cox, L. A., & Popken, D. A. (2014). Quantitative assessment of human MRSA risks from swine. *Risk Analysis, 34*(9), 1639–1650.

Danish Agriculture & Food Council. (2015). Statistics 2014—Pigmeat, Copenhagen.

Danmap. (2015). *Danmap 2014—Use of antimicrobial agents and occurence of antimicrobal resistance in bacteria from food animals and humans in Denmark, Copenhagen.*

DANMAP. (2016). *Use of antimicrobial agents and occurence of antimicrobial resistance in bacteria from food animals, food and humans in Denmark*. Report, November 2016. National Food Institute, Technical University of Denmark & Statens Serum Institut.

Deiters, C., Günnewig, V., Friedrich, A. W., Mellmann, A., & Köck, R. (2015). Are areas of methicillin-resistant *Staphylococcus aureus* clonal complex (CC) 398 among humans still livestock-associated? *International Journal of Medical Microbiology, 305*, 110–113.

Dixon, B. (1996). Killer bug ate my face. *Current Biology, 6*(5), 493.

Goffman, E. (1963). *Stigma: Notes on the management of spoiled identity*. Englewood Cliffs, NJ: Prentice-Hall Inc.

Herek, G. M., Gillis, J. R., & Cogan, J. C. (2009). Internalized stigma among sexual minority adults: Insights from a social psychological perspective. *Journal of Counseling Psychology, 56*(1), 32–43.

Köck, R., Schaumburg, F., Mellmann, A., et al. (2013). Livestock-associated methicillin-resistant *Staphylococcus aureus* (MRSA) as causes of human infection and colonization in Germany. *PLoS One, 8*(2), 1–6.

Link, B. G. (1987). Understanding labelling effects in the area of mental disorders: An assessment of the effects of expectations of rejection. *American Sociological Review, 52*(1), 96–112.

Link, B. G., & Phelan, J. C. (2001). Conceptualizing stigma. *Annual Review of Sociology, 27*, 363–385.

Livingston, J. D., & Boyd, J. E. (2010). Correlates and consequences of internalized stigma for people living with mental illness: A systematic review and meta-analysis. *Social Science & Medicine, 71*, 2150–2161.

National Board of Health. (2016). Information om MRSA af svinetype [Information about swine-related MRSA]. Online brief from https://sundhedsstyrelsen.dk, National Board of Health, Copenhagen, May 2016.

Statens Serum Institut. (2014). MRSA CC398-epidemiologien i Danmark, EPI-NYT, Copenhagen.

van Cleef, B. A., Verkade, E. J. M., Wulf, M. W., Buiting, A. G., Voss, A., et al. (2010). Prevalence of livestock-associated MRSA in communities with high pig-densities in The Netherlands. *PLoS ONE, 5*(2), e9385. https://doi.org/10.1371/journal.pone.0009385

9

What is 'Good Doctoring' When Antibiotic Resistance is a Global Threat?

Inge Kryger Pedersen and Kim Sune Jepsen

9.1 Introduction: Prevention of Antimicrobial Resistance as a New Jurisdictional Task

As a contribution to the field of sociological studies on professions and risks, this chapter lays out some results from an exploratory enquiry into 'good doctoring' in the case of antibiotic prescriptions. It is examined how general practitioners (GPs) govern and control current prescription practice in Danish primary care and how notions of 'good doctoring' may be relevant to understanding the practical handling and care of patients. In particular, this chapter explores the changing jurisdictions (Abbott 1988, 2005) of doctors and the transformative mechanisms that enable change to occur in clinical practice. In his seminal work on

I. K. Pedersen (✉)
Department of Sociology, University of Copenhagen, Copenhagen, Denmark
e-mail: ikp@soc.ku.dk

K. S. Jepsen
Department of Sociology, Lund University, Lund, Sweden
e-mail: kim_sune.jepsen@soc.lu

C. S. Jensen et al. (eds.), *Risking Antimicrobial Resistance*,
https://doi.org/10.1007/978-3-319-90656-0_9

professions, the American sociologist Andrew Abbott defines 'jurisdiction' as being the 'link between a profession and its work' (Abbott 1988, p. 20), whereby this chapter's objective is to contribute insights into new jurisdictional tasks in a risky environment. The focus will be on the challenges inherent in such a task, 'prevention of antimicrobial resistance', which are related not only to individual patients' health problems but also to global ones. It is demonstrated how GPs manage dilemmas in clinical practice if and when decisions about antibiotic prescriptions cannot be based on facts about molecular conditions. In this light, the chapter seeks to identify how GPs understand and evaluate jurisdictional boundaries, that is, how they control and apply their expert knowledge in regard to the public health issue of antibiotic resistance.

First, the theoretical, conceptual, and methodological framework will be specified. Second, a section of analysis combined with discussion, 'From commons to dual technologies', will provide insights into practices, tasks, and approaches of relevance to the antimicrobial resistance (AMR) problem as related to a range of tensions in clinical practice. This section contains four subsections. The first focuses on GPs' prescription practice and experiences seen against the background of a recent surveillance in Denmark showing a considerable increase in the total consumption of antibiotics in primary care within the last decade. The second subsection analyzes and discusses the general challenge of the 'One Health' perspective. The third subsection addresses how 'good doctoring' also involves handling tensions between guidelines and practice when global problems are translated into a clinical locality of consultation and medical expert practice. The last subsection points to essential tensions between different forms of medical knowledge relevant to the AMR problem, in particular the tension between epidemiology and pathophysiology. In the final section, it is concluded that conditions for defending 'prevention of antimicrobial resistance' as a prestigious and untouchable jurisdictional task are currently not available. It is emphasized that the broader external forces of global AMR must be seen as shaping medical practice in the locations of primary care.

9.2 Risky Doctoring and Working Jurisdictions

AMR poses considerable dangers to public health if even simple infections cannot be cured (WHO 2014) and the medical profession risks losing one of its most important tools in clinical practice. The AMR problem is one of very few exceptions where 'the global public', such as the World Health Organization (WHO) and the European Commission (EC), is interfering with and more or less explicitly questioning professional authority as a source of monopolizing treatment decisions. In this regard, AMR differs from most other pandemics because the development of antibiotics marks a form of progress in medical technology that is supposed to yield benefits but also carries unintended detrimental outcomes. AMR has arisen owing to medically produced circumstances linked to the excessive use of antibiotics (Aabenhus et al. 2016, p. 1; see also Beck 1992, pp. 204–212, for other examples of secondary consequences of medical progress). When medical technologies are problematized, in this case when, 'Excessive and inappropriate use of antibiotics is considered to be the most important driver of the development of resistance' (Aabenhus et al. 2016, p. 1), there may be consequences for clinical work even if AMR is not traceable to the personal practice of the individual doctor.

The German sociologist Ulrich Beck's risk perspective (1992) is a broader framework for bringing risk thinking into this chapter. He has argued that we live in a risk society where risks are constructed not least by expert systems. Risks do not refer to an experienced reality but to probabilities or, in Beck's approach, to possible societal scenarios, and our study is about how GPs handle a specific global scenario. In collaboration with Giddens and Lash, Beck has characterized so-called reflexive modernization (Beck et al. 1994), thus casting light on a general approach to authority. As Larsen has put it in an article about challenged authority in doctor-patient relationships, '...reflexive modernization can undermine our belief in authority, but at the same time increase the number and complexity of situations in which individuals need to depend upon specialized expertise' (Larsen 2016, p. 2).

On a practical level, the consequences of certain risks may be that individuals, whether doctors or patients, make choices and act—or not—based on worst-case scenarios and unknown threats that may concern them at some point in the future. In the case of AMR, the decision not to prescribe antibiotics when the doctor is in doubt that they will help the patient is part of such a consideration by which doctors seek to handle different risk realities.

Beck's discussion of 'risk society' is important to understanding that newly manufactured risks like AMR increasingly depend on specialized expert knowledge and its divergent problem scenarios and knowledge claims of what risks entail as well as how and by whom they must be tackled. From this perspective, we can see global threats like AMR as an emerging risks reality that is becoming increasingly contested by scientific expertise but also might feed into new uncertainties and doubts about who to believe in defining the AMR problem-solutions and who might bear responsibility for tackling this global risk.

While focusing on a medical subprofession, that of GPs, we seek to demonstrate the complex settlement of such difficult problems. As we suggest, the professional concerns informing how GPs handle the potentially global risk of AMR through their active negotiation of standards, guidelines, and situated prescription dilemmas demonstrate various manners of carrying out different modes of 'good doctoring'. That is, to underline that we are dealing with clinical practice, this chapter draws on the term 'doctoring' defined as 'the mode of knowing and acting specific to the clinic' (Struhkamp et al. 2009, p. 57). The issue we wish to address is thus the different modes of knowing, valuing, and acting by which GPs take control of their professional arena when treating diseases in view of a global risk reality such as AMR. Hence, questioning what good doctoring means when antibiotic resistance is a global threat, we follow Beck's suggestion that it is crucial and necessary to expose how specialized professional expertise operates in situations of uncertainty, not least by linking professional practice to its wider societal implications. In this regard, Beck has underlined the following: 'Medicine alone possesses in the form of the clinic an organizational arrangement in which development and application of research results to patients can be carried out and perfected autonomously and according to its own standards and categories in isolation from outside questions and monitoring' (Beck 1992, p. 210).

In particular, our exploration demonstrates how GPs handle antibiotic prescriptions in their clinical context, which is not discrete from wider societal and political interference in a global AMR risk reality. Hence, if Beck provides a lucid background for understanding AMR as an emerging global risk reality that implies new tasks of experts and forms of expertise in a reflexive process of modernization, then the following questions present themselves: how do global risk realities such as AMR become locally embedded in professional settlements, and how can such settlements be seen to entail different knowledge claims and practices, that is, what we have determined to be 'good doctoring'. In this regard, questions pertaining to doctors' authority and autonomy are part of the classic repertoires in research by the sociological profession. A claimed right stated by medical associations is that 'no third parties'—for example, governments or corporations and private companies—should erode professional authority by interfering with doctors' decision-making on behalf of their patients (Larsen 2016, p. 3). When political claims are made, such as those by transnational organizations and national health authorities, they may impinge on professional tasks and practice, jurisdictions, and visions. Prescriptions of antibiotics are not simply a matter of the doctors' making judgments and decisions. There are tensions between standards, regulations, and in particular, between guidelines and clinical 'reality'. Thus, dilemmas may be engendered by political claims (Pedersen and Jepsen 2018). In this chapter, we go deeper into such tensions by exploring what makes for good doctoring when guidelines are not or cannot be strictly followed.

In order to expose how the problem of antibiotic usage is understood and engaged with by GPs, we follow significant strands within the sociology of professions by drawing on Abbott's work on this subject. Instead of 'groups' of professions, Abbott focuses on how 'tasks and problems' are part of defining the executive boundaries of an expert specialty denoting authority, thus composing a jurisdiction. Abbott's definition opens the way to exploring how professionals actually *work* by setting up dynamic boundaries based on control via knowledge and practical tasks that need to be deemed *legitimate* by others: '…to perform skilled acts and justify them cognitively is not yet to hold jurisdiction. In claiming jurisdiction, a profession asks society to recognize its cognitive structure through exclusive rights; jurisdiction has not only a culture, but also a social structure' (Abbott 1988, p. 59).

If the capacities to define problems and perform legitimate skilled tasks demarcate a jurisdiction, Abbott's later work especially has made it clear that jurisdictions are dynamically linked through professional struggles of social control within their work area (Abbott 2005, p. 247). Social control of medical practice is in particular about securing the jurisdictional core task. That is, to cure remains only one important aspect of how jurisdictions work and what is at stake in maintaining them. We have found that an informal knowledge culture and clinical etiquettes are also important components when handling prescriptions of antibiotics (Pedersen and Jepsen 2018). In addition, the practical tasks of handling a disease are in the clinical context a substantial part of what makes up the jurisdictional boundaries and how risk realities are managed. That is to say, jurisdictions are not made up purely of 'social stuff' such as identities, issues of control and authority, but also of the normative conflicts that unfold around how a disease and the risk associated with actual antibiotic treatments play out among professional occupations, patients, standards, guidelines, measurement, and diagnostic tests and techniques.

If we translate the above theoretical concepts of jurisdiction, good doctoring and risk realities into the context of GPs' clinical work, we are obliged to consider antibiotic usage as a matter of 'how jurisdictions work', that is, how the boundaries of professional working areas are regulated (Abbott 1988, 2005). Abbott's view of jurisdictions not only links to 'closure' and inter-professional competitions but is also open-ended. He approaches jurisdictions as dynamic 'problem-spaces', in particular by means of his 'linked ecologies' perspective (2005). In line with this, the next section of analysis and discussion will demonstrate how the 'prevention of AMR' works as a jurisdictional task when clinical complexity interferes with rules set out by another body, for example, with *Danish Medical Society for General Practice* (DSAM) guidelines established by the GPs' own scientific society. However, prevention of AMR as a new task does not provoke a fight for jurisdiction on all levels. As Abbott himself emphasizes, intra- and inter-professional competition 'can be in many dimensions, over many things, with many different groups' (Abbott 2005, p. 3). Thus, this approach arguably allows for registering new tensions at work: uncertainties, ambiguities, or controversies between what is valued and how things are done; just as we allow GPs to delineate and position themselves in the social landscape of other professionals and pressing concerns in the antibiotic field. We have sought therefore to acquire knowledge of different normative registers of valuations that sustain professional jurisdictions and make it possible to look more closely at the open question, 'What is good doctoring?'

On this basis, we suggest that the jurisdictional task of 'prescribing antibiotics' is currently accompanied by that of 'prevention of antimicrobial resistance'. Or we can ask: which profession wants to claim this task? 'Professions develop when jurisdictions become vacant', Abbott says (Abbott 1988, p. 3). A vacant jurisdiction can be newly created or it can be abandoned or lost by another profession (Ibid.). 'Prevention of AMR' is globally a newly created jurisdictional task and will be explored as a transnational task that is likely changing intra- and inter-professional conditions and relations. When the jurisdiction includes global problems, doctoring might imply modes of knowing and acting from outside the clinic as well. The way 'doctoring' enacts AMR as risk realities will demonstrate how the AMR jurisdiction works. Hence, by using Abbott's suggestions, this chapter focuses on knowledge garnered from individual doctors' professional experience more than on science-based knowledge, which is Beck's primary source for his arguments in favor of risk politics based on reflexive accommodation between these two forms of knowledge (Beck 1992, pp. 223–235).

In line with our methodological focus on how good doctoring takes place within GPs' jurisdictional work, the study does not attempt to provide a representative picture of how the medical profession as a whole understands and engages with antibiotic usage in Denmark or elsewhere. Adopting a qualitative approach, we are concerned with exploring how a range of dilemmas and problems assert themselves in GPs' clinical practice and to address issues of good doctoring in line with our theoretical position. Very little is known about how doctors respond to global health problems in clinical practice. Interviewing provides access to such insights, exploring: (a) how GPs engage with knowledge, skills, and concrete tasks, for example, how they define and seek to apply antibiotics in the treatment of respiratory tract infections; and (b) how GPs understand and form opinions about the (global) health issue of antibiotic resistance. In conjunction, another objective is to explore and discuss the more structural transformations that general practice presumably is undergoing in respect to new guidelines, policies, scientific advice, and concerns within the field of diagnosing and prescribing antibiotics in light of the AMR risk.

Empirical materials include documents (reports from WHO, EC, DANMAP [*The Danish Integrated Antimicrobial Resistance Monitoring and Research Program*], standard procedures, guidelines, and registration forms) and qualitative in-depth interviews with 21 GPs, as well as meetings with key persons about goals, dilemmas and practices. In order to explore the research questions, this paper draws mainly on literature and the interview material, where documents are used as background. The interviewees were selected with a view to ensure as broad a range as possible in terms of gender, age, geographical location, and occupational experience. As an offshoot of this sampling strategy, we pursued in particular an interest in different occupational experiences linked to forms of practice: solo as well as collaborative practices (for more about methods and methodological considerations, see Pedersen and Jepsen 2018, pp. 4–6).

9.3 From Commons to Dual Technologies

The title of this section signals a general tension that has appeared within the last decades since AMR has become a widespread problem. Before then, antibiotics were recognized almost exclusively as a common good, whereas currently there is more awareness that they also can harm by creating bacterial resistance. Based on all our material, including relevant studies and literature, we have selected four significant relations to be discussed when GPs negotiate jurisdictional tasks. These relations entail surveillances and GPs' experiences; One Health and GPs' core task; guidelines and clinical practice; epidemiology and pathophysiology. By providing topics and examples, we will illustrate how 'good doctoring' in the informal arena of the workplace (Abbott 1988, p. 60, 66)—here clinical practice—might differ from what is recognized as 'good doctoring' in the formal arenas of the public and legal realms (Ibid., pp. 60–69). Therefore, 'relations' sometimes should be understood as 'tensions'. Since this chapter is short and AMR is a recognized problem, the focus will be on the latter rather than on non-conflictual relations. In what follows, the discussion of tensions takes as its point of theoretical departure Abbott's distinctions between formal arenas and the informal arena that is clinical practice.

9.3.1 Surveillances and GPs' Experiences

The Danish Integrated Antimicrobial Resistance Monitoring and Research Program, DANMAP, started in 1995 and its recent surveillance has shown an increase within primary care of about 20 percent from 2004 to 2013, herein a 72 percent increase in the use of broad-spectrum antibiotics (DANMAP 2013, p. 15). As we were interviewing the GPs and we presented these findings about the consumption of antibiotics in Denmark, almost all of the interviewees expressed surprise. Indeed, this considerable increase did not correspond to most of the GPs' perceptions and they did not assume that they themselves had prescribed more and more antibiotics. Quite a few knew about other doctors' prescribing antibiotics in more situations than they themselves would do. However, it was not considered suitable to interfere. As one of the GPs said, 'No, there's a kind of inappropriateness around that. You can't make it an issue (…) I would feel then that I was claiming myself to be better acquainted with our field, which might not be the case. It's about a form of collegiality in some way' (GP10).

In an article about 'non-medical issues' related to prescriptions of antibiotics, this chapter's authors have illustrated how professional etiquette ensures that doctors in general do not interfere in peers' assessments and practices (Pedersen and Jepsen 2018, pp. 9–10). Likewise, when interviewing eighty GPs in the UK, Armstrong & Ogden found that by using mechanisms of etiquette, the GPs would seek to secure clinical autonomy (2006, p. 955).

Some of the GPs in our study had acquired insights into their own clinic's prescription pattern by gaining access to medical advisers' comparisons to other—anonymous and comparable—clinics. In such measures, they did not perceive a loss of autonomy or control. As Weiss and Fitzpatrick also found in their study based on interviews with medical advisers and GPs in the UK, GPs' concern about external control was 'more a concern that too inflexible an approach would limit their use of prescribing as a pragmatic problem-solving device' (Weiss and Fitzpatrick 1997, p. 314). GPs in our study described how such surveillances had changed their assumptions about their own or the whole clinic's prescription pattern. One of them said, 'We wouldn't let [our past prescription pattern] hang over our heads. He [the medical adviser] came the next year, and at that time, we were below [the average]' (GP1). The GPs with such experiences found those ways of getting information appropriate—and provocative—as well as offering a learning dimension without violating the clinical etiquette. Thévenot has termed these kinds of activities a set of compromises that 'manages the tension between standardization requirements and the decentralization of local practices' (2001, p. 417). In the section 'Guidelines and Clinical Practice', we further explore such tensions.

A significant difference in prescription patterns might be related to the 'ideology' of younger doctors who are more likely to follow medical standards than their older colleagues, some of the GPs said. For example, this was touched upon by one of the younger GPs in the following way: 'I think that as a young doctor you're almost ideological, I was about to say. We're certainly brought up with the problem of antibiotic resistance and I believe that I'm very strict compared with my older colleagues (…) I always start with narrow-spectrum antibiotics' (GP6).

Another young GP asserted that more experienced GPs might build their potentially more generous dispensing of antibiotics upon important and sometimes also bad experiences (GP3). Several of the more experienced GPs' accounts confirmed that safety was an important reason for prescribing antibiotics:

> The first patient I saw today got antibiotics (…) He wasn't terribly sick (…) that is, he wasn't suffering from a high fever and wasn't that bad. When I

> take a decision like this and choose to prescribe antibiotics, I do it in light of what's happened before (...) Last time he was sick, he was hospitalized, so I didn't have the courage not to prescribe antibiotics. I could have performed a blood test to support my decision, but I don't think I would have changed my mind because he isn't that resilient and he's 78 years old (...) you lower the bar when you've had bad experiences. (GP1)

The surveillances should have indicated a decrease in prescriptions if younger generations of doctors in general and throughout their career have become stricter about prescribing broad-spectrum antibiotics. Indeed, all the GPs suggested several other explanations for the increased use of antibiotics, and taken all together, these accounts provided a complex and multifaceted explanation. Other explanations suggested were, for example, attributed to the growing prevalence of COPD (Chronic Obstructive Pulmonary Disease) and a relatively older population. All GPs had experiences of prescribing antibiotics for safety reasons. Antibiotic prophylaxis refers to the use of antibiotics to prevent infection, that is, in cases like those of COPD patients, to prevent worse ill health. Another explanation was related to a health political discourse of limiting as much as possible the number of patients admitted to hospital.

A general issue mentioned by almost all GPs was worried and stressful parents of small kids and how day-care centers sometimes demanded that kids should be receiving treatment, if not, staying at home. GP9 gave a kind of 'ecological' explanation related to how busier working conditions in different settings might feed into one another: GPs have got less time for each patient; many patients also are busy at work and have no time for sick leave; at the day-care centers, more and more children have to be squeezed together and there is not much time for outside activities, which means that they get sick more often; employees at the day-care service have less time to take care of kids feeling bad, so they phone parents promptly; parents get stressed, and so on. Such 'non-medical issues' (see also Lundkvist et al. 2002; Stivers 2007) may result in more antibiotics being prescribed, although all those involved are doing their work and providing the best care possible. While they might not conform to what the surveillances show longitudinally, GPs do experience tensions and changes, possibly indicating awareness of the excessive use of antibiotics as a risk.

9.3.2 One Health and GPs' Core Task

When we asked our interviewees questions to enhance our understanding of 'good doctoring', they did not just evaluate their practice and knowledge, but also reflected upon current situations in the labor market, as we saw above. Furthermore, they told us about what they and their colleagues or others, for example, vets or the *Danish Health Authorities*, might do—or were not able to do—to improve practice and knowledge. This part of dealing with their experiences also emphasizes that the GPs do not act alone. Indeed, this is an important reason why we focus on 'good doctoring', instead of 'perfect doctoring'. The GPs are able to evaluate their practice as good or bad from the perspective of what is possible when they do not act alone but in conjunction with lots of people, professions, guidelines, diagnostic tests, health politics and institutions—not to mention bacteria.

It should be emphasized that all GPs more or less explicitly expressed that 'good doctoring' is first and foremost about taking care of the individual patient. As one of them said, 'I think—to hit the nail on the head—that the care of the individual patient must prevail in the end, compared with antibiotic issues on the national or global level. However, it [prescription of antibiotics] ought to be handled in a very rational way' (GP10).

The general core task of medical doctors as a profession is to cure. However, in GPs' clinical practice, the core task is, in a broader sense, to take care of the individual patient. With all that this implies, cure and care can create 'good doctoring'. To cure is a more evident core task of other medical specialties and GPs may position themselves differently, as we will see below, when it comes to tensions between guidelines and clinical practice, which include intra- and inter-professional tensions. For the purpose of 'reducing the use of antimicrobials as much as possible and to maximize coordinated efforts between the human health sector and the veterinary sector in the fight against AMR' (EC 2012, p. 2), the One Health perspective can be seen as an attempt by external forces not only to avoid inter-professional contests, but also to mobilize absorption of AMR within the internal structure of existing professions in the hope of more effective results. The GPs' accounts also express that the develop-

ment—and the prevention—of AMR is born out of social circumstances within the human, as well as the veterinary, domain.

Some GPs emphasized that the problem mainly results from developments within agriculture. For example, one of the GPs said: 'The [vets] use it [antibiotics] as population-prophylaxis where "the population" is in this instance the whole pig population. The pigs get it in their feedstuff. It corresponds to adding antibiotics to cornflakes [breakfast cereal] for human populations with many cases of otitis' (GP1).

Challenges to clinical practice posed by external forces in the form of political developments, One Health perspectives, and new scientific developments may not constrain GPs to change their behavior. Guidelines were literally considered guidelines and not directives. None of the interviewees addressed the AMR problem in a way as if no changes at all were needed to escape the worst-case scenario: that antibiotics become a useless tool in clinical practice. Some GPs believed that the AMR challenge should be resolved by others and in other areas, in particular within agriculture, and at other levels such as policy. Moreover, they sought more scientific knowledge of how best to handle the AMR problem.

9.3.3 Guidelines and Clinical Practice

From the GPs' accounts, it appears that daily practices sometimes are compatible with guidelines, whereas sometimes they clash. However, guideline recommendations for prescription of antibiotics did not seem to command much attention among most of the interviewees, and none of the GPs' DGEs (groups of 10–15 peers that meet regularly about medical issues) had put the antibiotic issue on their meeting agendas. Other issues seemed more urgent, the GPs told us. Based on literature reviews about the usefulness, as well as the effectiveness, of guidelines in general, Timmermans and Kolker have concluded that guidelines do not seem to change practice significantly, but they are good to have—for doctors and their organizations, as well as patients, biomedical researchers, governments agencies, and policymakers (2004, pp. 182–183). From our interview accounts, we can recognize what Woolf et al. (1999, p. 528) state about guidelines: 'They offer explicit recommendations for clinicians who are uncertain about how to proceed, overturn the beliefs of doctors accustomed to outdated practices, improve the consistency of care, and provide authoritative recommendations that reassure practitioners about the appropriateness of their treatment policies'.

However, as Timmermans and Kolker put it: 'If educational insights would be the only benefit of clinical practice guidelines, they would never have received the attention and resources they command today' (2004, p. 182). GPs in our study emphasized their use of guidelines as a tool, sometimes to improve the quality of clinical decisions, but mostly to confirm what they had assessed themselves. In acute consultations for assessing possible infections, short guidelines were preferred. Most importantly—and this is actually what all the tensions discussed here are about—the GPs underlined by several concrete examples that local needs could be rather different from what is prescribed by guidelines across sites. One of the GPs said, '… our guidelines are more and more created by people who are not familiar with our daily situations, (…) for example, by ear-nose-throat specialists, who have a professional focus on a selected subpopulation of children with ear disorders' (GP5).

This concern indicated another tension as well, namely, that although doctors produce guidelines for doctors, often doctors within other specialties are involved in creating the guidelines and sometimes their suggestions are far from the reality of clinical practice.

Many research projects and much literature have tried suggesting new strategies for helping to disseminate more appropriate treatment advice to change professional practice, in particular with respect to better guidelines (e.g., Lugtenberg et al. 2009). The GPs' own scientific society, DSAM, has in light of the AMR problem recently developed comprehensive clinical guidelines for antibiotic prescriptions. Guidelines embody the extent of medicine's jurisdiction (Timmermans and Kolker 2004, p. 178) and are a means of controlling professional knowledge and its application (Abbott 1988, p. 2). Very few, however, have tried to identify *why* many of these strategies, for example, dissemination of information, did not seem to change professional practice (Armstrong and Ogden 2006; Bero et al. 1998). This fact has indeed led us to conduct our study, and the analysis and discussion in this subsection has demonstrated how the jurisdiction and 'internal forces' can work when clinical complexity interferes with the knowledge base of guidelines. In what follows, we will discuss another tension that seems to be active and relevant to address when examining clinical complexity.

9.3.4 Epidemiology and Pathophysiology

GPs deal with risks, indeed at a level other than risk management in the formal arenas. Timmermans and Kolker's key finding is that guidelines constitute a shift in the medical knowledge base, namely from pathophysiology to epidemiology. As they argue: 'The randomized clinical trial has replaced the autopsy as the gold standard in medicine, and it has consolidated a quantitative, population-based way of looking at health and illness' (2004, p. 182). The new evidence-based medical paradigm assumes that 'an understanding of pathophysiology is necessary but insufficient for the practice of clinical medicine' (Ibid.). The effectiveness of all kinds of interventions, whether diagnostic or therapeutic, should have been demonstrated by means of robust empirical studies. Pathophysiology is still of great importance and 'necessary', and medical doctors' professional power is intact. However, within formal arenas, at 'a broader political-organizational level', as Timmermans and Kolker put it (Ibid., p. 183), the turn toward statistics and population health involves a shift in how to research and intervene in health from the individual to the aggregate level (Hacking 1990; see also Wahlberg and Rose 2015).

In this light, Timmermans and Kolker discuss how the control over professional knowledge might change and they emphasize the importance of a specific question: who creates guidelines (2004, pp. 184ff)? As we have illustrated above, indeed there are some tensions between guidelines and clinical practice, also with reference to the creators of the guidelines. Most of the interviewees even prefer to use guidelines other than those created by their own scientific society, and quite a few are not aware of the most recent guideline recommendations by DSAM. Such preferences and practices might be related to the general discussion about what 'evidence-based knowledge' is and means, both within medicine and other professional areas as well (see, e.g., Sackett et al. 1996). This discussion is essential to an understanding of intra-professional changes.

Yet, as Timmermans and Kolker state, these changes have escaped much of 'contemporary theorizing on the medical profession' (2004, p. 184).

Sociological and cognate social science studies have been more focused on the role of guidelines and how, rather than why, they have not succeeded in becoming an effective policy tool. In the medical science literature, the focus has been mostly on the standardizing form of practice guidelines (Ibid., p. 186). Our study and others have demonstrated how guidelines seem to create some tensions in clinical practice, in particular between a clinic's specific local cases or situations and guidelines for use across clinics (e.g., Armstrong and Ogden 2006; Pedersen and Jepsen 2018; Woolf et al. 1999). In daily practice, clinical autonomy and discretionary powers might still 'attenuate the standardizing forces', as indicated by our study, as well as Timmermans and Kolker's study of asthma guidelines and literature reviews. A deeper investigation probably would turn up something to do with the tensions between different forms of medical knowledge, all of which are very important but maybe within different levels and arenas. In Chap. 11 we will follow up on this topic by presenting different political and moral regimes for justifying issues related to antibiotics; the discussion supplements this chapter by digging deeper for explanations as to *why* tensions and dilemmas can arise when doctors handle prescriptions for antibiotics.

'Good doctoring' is inscribed with such tensions. Standardizations ensure a spatial equivalence across clinics and sometimes transnationally. However, yielding to the patients' demands or needs, and maybe experiencing a shortage of time, undermines the guidelines' requirements of regularity, stabilization, and standardization. The decisions made by GPs may be compromised also by patients' freedom to choose another practitioner. In the case of AMR, at least in Denmark, GPs may be less focused on patients' being attracted by other GPs than on their more easily accessing antibiotics elsewhere, which some GPs mention as an important factor in their decision-making.

To sum up, a tension between different kinds of medical knowledge can be activated by new epidemiological findings and may originate in the reality that discretion in clinical practice requires formal tools such as guidelines (Timmermans and Kolker 2004, pp. 188–189). If medical knowledge—and power—also consists in creating a productive doctor-patient encounter, involving patients, listening to and teaching them to secure adherence, taking into consideration financial and time pressures and lots of other things, which some GPs call 'non-medical issues', then this term is misleading. Such issues must also be considered medical if guidelines and other standardizing tools work in practice and are not just sometimes-forgotten formalities distant from the realities of the profession. This is where conceiving of professions as living in an ecology (Abbott 1988) opens up a dynamic view on what creates professional boundaries. Indeed, all the aforementioned issues are taken into account in 'good doctoring', although they are situated at the boundaries of medical jurisdiction. Not every task is or can be tightly structured, and so GPs, by bringing their force to bear on many different issues, also provide strength, intra- as well as inter-professionally.

9.4 Conclusion and Perspectives: 'Good Doctoring' Is Handling Tensions

The risks of prescribing antibiotics might not refer directly to an experienced reality. They are instead 'man-made hybrids' to cite Ulrich Beck (1992, p. 221)—hybrids based on expectations and 'calculations' of potentialities and probabilities. The decision not to prescribe antibiotics when the doctor is in doubt about whether they will help the patient is part of such considerations by which doctors handle different risk realities. More research is needed into what kinds of risk realities are managed. Yet this chapter has demonstrated the risk context in which GPs operate when stating that use of antibiotics might imply health risks at a (global) population level. Clinical practice may differ from the imperatives of the risk discourse. The surveillances, as well as the dilemmas and the narratives from the clinics, tell us that it does. The GPs' accounts have demonstrated that the health risks in not prescribing antibiotics if they later turn out to be necessary weigh heavily in certain situations.

The specific situations of handling antibiotic use and antimicrobial resistance should not be reduced to how medical professions orient themselves toward internal situations. The broader external forces of global AMR, the development of international and national policies and guidelines, as well as the jurisdictional claims of other professions, must be seen as a part of shaping medical practice in the locations of primary care. Current studies suggest that overprescription might be a common phenomenon that relates to organizational pressures, misguided expectations, and a concern for safety that would appear to contradict the guidelines for 'prudent use'. This chapter has demonstrated that to explore how 'good doctoring' is handled in clinical practice entails a focus on controversial situations and normative concerns in managing tensions within four relations: Surveillances and GPs' experiences; One Health and GPs' core task; guidelines and clinical practice; epidemiology and pathophysiology. These are relations that GPs themselves have touched upon to account for their actions, and they seem an appropriate basis from which to proceed, with further research focusing on explanations of professional practice other than those based only on provision of knowledge.

The manner in which antibiotics as a common good is differently qualified and engaged with by professionals, here GPs, has become a focal point in view of increasing resistance. The analysis and discussion have suggested that the phenomenon of overprescription raises significant questions to be explored. To explain how global problems are (or sometimes are not) translated into consultation and clinical practice, further research must be conducted to disclose how medico ideas feed into the policy process and how governance networks are linked. Although GPs in many countries, indeed in Denmark itself, control the prescribing of antibiotics, practitioners may be subject to guidelines from their own scientific society; for instance, the DSAM took the initiative of creating new guidelines, indicating that GPs may still have to contend with jurisdictional control issues. As Abbott has stated, the prestige of a professional knowledge system is connected to the ability of the profession to keep and defend its jurisdiction. Moreover, the more logical, scientific, and rigorous the knowledge system, the more prestigious and untouchable the jurisdiction: 'criteria of success may vary with task', as he says (1988, p. 104). Currently, the transnational jurisdictional task of 'prevention of antimicrobial resistance' seems defended at the organizational level. Only by studying workplaces, in this case clinical practices, can we acquire knowledge about the way in which professional jurisdictional tasks are enacted. Furthermore, we need additional examinations and empirical testing of transnational professional issues not just among professions involved in the AMR problem but also across political and university ecologies.

References

Aabenhus, R., Siersma, V., Hansen, M. P., & Bjerrum, L. (2016). Antibiotic prescribing in Danish general practice 2004–2013. *Journal of Antimicrobial Chemotherapy, 71*(8), 2286–2294.

Abbott, A. (1988). *The system of professions: An essay on the division of expert labor*. Chicago: University of Chicago Press.

Abbott, A. (2005). Linked ecologies: States and universities as environments for professions. *Sociological Theory, 23*(3), 245–274.

Armstrong, D., & Ogden, J. (2006). The role of etiquette and experimentation in explaining how doctors change behaviour: A qualitative study. *Sociology of Health & Illness, 28*(7), 951–968.

Beck, U. (1992). *Risk society. Towards a new modernity*. London: Sage Publications.

Beck, U., Giddens, A., & Lash, S. (1994). *Reflexive modernization. politics, tradition and aesthetics in the modern social order*. Cambridge: Polity Press.

Bero, L. A., Grilli, R., Grimshaw, J. M., Harvey, E., Oxman, A. D., & Thomson, M. A. (1998). Getting research findings into practice: Closing the gap between research and practice: An overview of systematic reviews of interventions to promote the implementation of research findings. *BMJ: British Medical Journal, 317*(7156), 465–468.

DANMAP. (2013). *DANMAP 2013—Use of antimicrobial agents and occurrence of antimicrobial resistance in bacteria from food animals, food and humans in Denmark*. The Danish Integrated Antimicrobial Resistance Monitoring and Research Program. Copenhagen: Statens Serum Institute.

EC. (2012). *Council conclusions on the impact of antimicrobial resistance in the human health sector and in the veterinary sector—A "One Health" perspective*. Brussels: The Council of the European Union.

Hacking, I. (1990). *The taming of chance*. Cambridge: Cambridge University Press.

Larsen, L. T. (2016). No third parties. The medical profession reclaims authority in doctor-patient relationships. *Professions & Professionalism, 6*(2), 1–14.

Lugtenberg, M., Zegers-van Schaick, J. M., Westert, G. P., & Burgers, J. S. (2009). Why don't physicians adhere to guideline recommendations in practice? An analysis of barriers among Dutch general practitioners. *Implementation Science, 4*(54), 1–8.

Lundkvist, J., Akerlind, I., Borgquist, L., & Mölstad, S. (2002). The more time spent on listening, the less time spent on prescribing antibiotics in general practice. *Family Practice, 19*(6), 638–640.

Pedersen, I. K., & Jepsen, K. S. (2018). Prescribing antibiotics: General practitioners dealing with "non-medical issues"? *Professions & Professionalism, 8*(1), 1–14.

Sackett, D. L., Rosenberg, W. M. C., Gray, J. A. M., Haynes, R. B., & Richardson, W. S. (1996). Evidence based medicine: What it is and what it isn't. *BMJ: British Medical Journal, 312*(7023), 71–72.

Stivers, T. (2007). *Prescribing under pressure: Parent-physician conversations and antibiotics*. Oxford: Oxford University Press.

Struhkamp, R., Mol, A., & Swierstra, T. (2009). Dealing with in/dependence. Doctoring in physical rehabilitation practice. *Science, Technology, & Human Values, 34*(1), 55–76.

Thévenot, L. (2001). Organized complexity. Conventions of coordination and the composition of economic arrangements. *European Journal of Social Theory, 4*(4), 405–425.

Timmermans, S., & Kolker, E. S. (2004). Evidence-based medicine and the reconfiguration of medical knowledge. *Journal of Health and Social Behavior, 45*(Suppl), 177–193.

Wahlberg, A., & Rose, N. (2015). The governmentalization of living: Calculating global health. *Economy and Society, 44*(1), 60–90.

Weiss, M., & Fitzpatrick, R. (1997). Challenges to medicine: The case of prescribing. *Sociology of Health & Illness, 19*(3), 297–327.

WHO. (2014). *Antimicrobial resistance: 2014 global report on surveillance*. Geneva: World Health Organization.

Woolf, S. H., Grol, R., Hutchinson, A., Eccles, M., & Grimshaw, J. (1999). Potential benefits, limitations, and harms of clinical guidelines. *BMJ: British Medical Journal, 318*(7182), 527–530.

10

Governing Risk by Conveying Just Enough (Un)Certainty: Rearticulating Good Doctoring as a Psy-Medical Competence

Mads Bank and Anne Rogne

10.1 Introduction

The primary care system is responsible for a vast majority of all prescriptions for antibiotics within the Danish healthcare system. Hence, primary care is an important site for understanding and developing interventions to promote responsible use of antibiotics. Within this field, it is widely acknowledged that Denmark, along with a few other countries, stands out in relation to antibiotic stewardship (Cordoba et al. 2015). In accordance with the common rationales within medicine and healthcare, this can be explained by a high level of knowledge among general practitioners (GPs), dispersion of knowledge through clinical

M. Bank (✉)
Department of Public Health, University of Copenhagen, Copenhagen, Denmark
e-mail: bank@madsbank.com

A. Rogne
'Psykologisk korttidsrådgivning' ('Psychological Counseling') Copenhagen, Copenhagen, Denmark
e-mail: anne.rogne@psy.ku.dk

C. S. Jensen et al. (eds.), *Risking Antimicrobial Resistance*,
https://doi.org/10.1007/978-3-319-90656-0_10

guidelines as well as a widespread use of point-of-care-tests (POCT). Nevertheless, it is still acknowledged that GPs regularly prescribe in ways that contradict knowledge of best practice and clinical guidelines (e.g. Jørgensen et al. 2013).

In the following chapter, we investigate this apparent discrepancy through an empirical study of how general practitioners diagnose and manage diseases that may result in a prescription of antibiotics.

The first part of the chapter presents an overview of the current research on unnecessary antibiotic prescription within general practice and how this problem is currently perceived and handled. We argue that a bio-medical logic focusing on knowledge dominates both research strategies and popular discourses about healthcare. We draw on anthropologist Annemarie Mol's concept of logic in order to show how clinical encounters about possible antibiotic prescription are not just about knowledge but also influenced and mediated by discursive, affective, psychological, cultural, and meaning-making processes. We believe that much research does not address the complexity of prescription behaviours and the clinical encounter because the bio-medical logic of medical practice and knowledge practices is in many instances sufficient to both understand and improve healthcare. However, problems arise when this logic, reproduced in current research strategies, becomes the sole model for how to understand healthcare. When knowledge becomes the dominant or only strategy for intervention, we become prone to engage in a perpetual race for more 'objective knowledge' which makes us blind to the complexity of what actually goes on in healthcare practices and other strategies of intervention.

In the second part of this chapter, we outline how our research strategy, inspired by Science and Technology Studies (STS), and in particular the work of Mol (2002, 2008), can avoid these pitfalls. In accordance with such an approach, our main interest has been to explore how clinical encounters regarding possible antibiotic prescription are handled by GPs and patients, and how meaning-making processes, different logics, and ways of thinking interact when various actors (GPs, patients, medication, machines, and so on) work together in order to improve a patient's situation.

In the third part of the chapter, we turn our attention to clinical encounters where the ubiquitous logic of (bio-medical) knowledge is less easily applied. We analyse cases where no clear-cut diagnosis, treatment, and prescription of antibiotics can be given, showing how such situations give rise to a characteristic state of uncertainty, or what we term 'liminal zones of uncertainty'. This allows us to investigate how the risk, uncertainty, and affective states implied in such 'zones' are addressed and responded to by the GP. Following this, we suggest the concept of 'psy-medical competence' as a broader interpretive frame when seeking to understand how GPs manage clinical encounters in ways that do not rely exclusively on knowledge.

Finally, we argue that this study will be of relevance in the fight against unnecessary prescription of antibiotics within general practice because it presents alternative frameworks for understanding and approaching consultations in which there is an insufficient number of indicators for treating a patient with an antibiotic.

In the conclusion, we broaden the scope of our study, discussing its relevance to how we 'educate' or govern subjects to be competent users of the healthcare system.

10.2 Research on Antibiotic Prescription in General Practice

The relatively low rate of antibiotics prescribed within the Nordic countries tends to be attributed to several factors, the most important being strict policy-making, a comprehensive use of clinical guidelines, and widespread availability of POCTs (e.g. Jakobsen et al. 2010; Jansbøl et al. 2012). Nevertheless, studies have shown that GPs still prescribe antibiotics in ways not always consistent with clinical guidelines, resulting in unnecessary prescribing of antibiotics and possible overprescribing (e.g. Jørgensen et al. 2013). The observed lack of adherence to evidence-based diagnostic and therapeutic knowledge has thus directed attention to what GPs know, how protocols are implemented, and to various barriers impeding adherence to the clinical guidelines (e.g. Grol et al. 2013). In fact, a number of qualitative studies have shown that GPs often prescribe antibiotics in *deliberate* inconsistency with current evidence-based recommendations, invoking contextual factors such as time pressure, perceived patient expectations, and a desire to maintain good relations (Ackerman et al. 2013; Hansen et al. 2015; Strandberg et al. 2013). Since unnecessary prescribing of antibiotics cannot solely be ascribed to a lack of knowledge (see also Stivers 2007), increased recognition must be given to the complexity of prescribing behaviour (Duane et al. 2016; Rodrigues et al. 2016). This complexity points to an urgent need to investigate the multiple influences on acting and thinking when it comes to prescription behaviour within clinical encounters (Cordoba et al. 2015; Gonzalez-Gonzalez et al. 2015). Thus, several papers have called for prevailing survey methods and research strategies to be supplemented by more qualitative studies and approaches (e.g. Tonkin-Crine et al. 2015), in order to identify the behavioural or psychological factors that underlie attitudes towards antibiotic prescribing (Cordoba et al. 2015) or gaps between the health-care system and professionals' knowledge and attitudes (Lopez-Vazquez et al. 2012).

What we will nevertheless argue is that such calls for alternative approaches to understanding prescription behaviour and explaining over-prescription continue to be haunted by a specific reasoning, dividing what happens in medical practices into two distinct 'realms'. In the work of Mol (2002), this approach is referred to as 'perspectivalism'. It is the task and privilege of biomedicine and its actors—natural scientists, practitioners, technologies, and textbooks—to tell the truth about, as well as study the physical reality of bodies and diseases; but it is nevertheless acknowledged that there is more to this world than that. Something has to be *added* to the physicalities that are the object of biomedicine. This 'something' consists of the meanings, the feelings, and the interpretations that accompany this physical reality when different actors approach it from various *perspectives*. Following such reasoning, studies of prescription behaviour can target either one of the two interlinked, but separate, realms. It can be a problem of what we *know*, that is, of the truth that has (or has not yet) been unveiled by those who study the reality of bacteria, infections, and antibiotics, or a problem of the knowledge that practitioners possess (or do not possess) *about* this reality. As demonstrated in, among others, the work of Timmermans and Berg (2003), this is the realm that is targeted when clinical guidelines are deployed in order to disseminate knowledge to assist practitioners in their decisions about the care of individual patients. And likewise, it is this realm that is targeted when qualitative studies make use of surveys and interviews to disclose what GPs *know* about current best evidence when making a decision about prescribing an antibiotic. Such reasoning nevertheless separates knowledge from the practicalities of what happens in the concrete encounter.

On the other hand, qualitative studies, as demonstrated, can acknowledge that prescription behaviour is modulated by more than sheer knowledge; that is, practitioners and patients might actually *know* better, but other factors nevertheless influence them to act contrary to such knowledge. One significant research tradition that seeks to understand these 'additional' influences on prescription behaviour is conversational analysis (CA). As an example, Stivers (2007) explores how different ways of presenting problems, questioning, and turn-taking cause GPs to experience being pressured into prescribing antibiotics, with the obvious risk of overprescribing. Stivers' analysis shows that what is most often at stake within these consultations is not a pressure for a prescription, but a wish for positive treatment recommendations, resolving the patient's discomfort and concerns while simultaneously legitimizing the visit to the GP. However, as Mol argues (2002), CA is still effective within the general scheme of perspectivalism. That is, even though it is acknowledged that both patients and doctors have a *perspective* and interpret the world they live in, the divide remains between the realm of the body's physical reality and the realm of meaning. As Mol (2002, p. 12) puts it, disease still '*recedes* behind the interpretations'. Mol sets herself the task of demonstrating how a closer look at the practices of diagnosing and treating disease shows us that the existence of this gap, again and again affirmed in the way we seek to both study and intervene in practice, is an analytical construction. She does this by showing how diseases are events-in-practice that are enacted through the cooperation of several people, through their actions as well as their words.

10.3 The Methodological and Theoretical Approach

In order to approach the field in a way that moves beyond the limitations inherent in prevailing methods and the gap between the body's physical reality and meaning attached to it that they enforce, we have therefore sought inspiration from the methods and concepts of the field of Science, Technology and Society (STS) studies. STS methods and concepts help us to design an explorative study that looks into the practicalities of caring for patients when they present themselves with a possible bacterial infection. As already mentioned, we have been particularly informed by the ethnographic studies of various health care practices by the anthropologist Annemarie Mol. Mol (2002) insists on a line of inquiry that she describes as 'praxiographical', referring to the attitude of stubbornly 'taking notice of the techniques that make things visible, audible, tangible, knowable' (p. 33), acknowledging that a disease never stands alone, but 'depends on everything and everyone that is active while it is being practiced' (p. 32). Furthermore, we follow Mol's approach (2008) in making the object of her inquires neither patients nor practitioners, but instead the practicalities of health care and the 'logics' immanent to them. According to Mol, the notion of 'logics' resembles the Foucauldian 'discourse', referring to the concrete formations of how 'words, materialities and practices hang together in a specific, historically and culturally situated way' (p. 9). Hence, she directs our attention to the rationality, or rationale inherent in any given practice, by which some ways of acting and thinking are deemed acceptable, desirable, or called for in a particular setting while other practices are stigmatized, repressed, or prevented. Such logics are not necessarily explicitly articulated, but rather embedded in practices. Doing praxiographical field work with attention to logics therefore requires that consultations must be observed and people interviewed, but such talk is not about the actors' knowledge nor opinions, but rather the events and activities observed and what rationalities as well as ideals that are embedded in and have inspired such specific ways of approaching and thinking about the care of patients with potential bacterial infections.

As such, we conducted two rounds of observations of clinical encounters in the practice of eight different GPs. These data then served as the platform for qualitative interviews with practitioners using stimulated recall to probe into the reasons, thoughts, and logics embedded in, as well as inspiring concrete care practices.

Going through our empirical material, we decided to narrow our analysis down to clinical encounters regarding a suspected respiratory infection. Besides taking its theoretical point of departure in the work of Mol, this analysis will draw upon research in the fields of medical anthropology (Timmermans and Berg 2003), psychology (Stenner and Moreno-Gabriel 2013), governmentality (Dean 1999), and affect studies (Massumi 1993).

10.4 Analysis: Rendering Suffering Knowable and Treatable

As we reviewed, coded, and analysed our data, we found that many of the observed encounters did not seem to be particularly surprising or problematic. They more or less followed the standard protocol for the decisions to be made about the care of a patient with a suspected respiratory infection; that is, we could observe the presence of various signs and symptoms affirmed prior to a POCT. The encounters followed the biomedical logic: a causal relationship between a bacterial or viral origin confined to a simple location and the reported symptoms, identified via the expertise and instruments of the GP. And when a POCT is applied and a visible line at the Strep A-test appears, a sufficient amount of indicators 'allows' for the prescription of an antibiotic. In such instances, particular parts of a patient's experience, together with the test results are abstracted from a complex reality and objectified in terms of a 'clear-cut' diagnosis referred to as 'bacterial pharyngitis'. Such consultations will most often go unnoticed since the production of an objective diagnosis makes the patient's suffering feasible, knowable, and treatable. As such, these are prototypical examples of the success of bio-medical logic and the practice based on such ideas.

We do not argue that specialized knowledge of biomedicine is a problem. The problem is rather a blindness to how a bio-medical logic produces a simplification (albeit successful), such that clinical encounters and lived reality are understood almost exclusively as a matter of knowledge, making it difficult to address and handle imprudent prescription behaviour through other strategies. Our aim, therefore, is to explore what is at stake when consultations are not easily resolved by producing objective bio-medical knowledge, and to analyse how such practices draw upon several intertwined and juxtaposed logics. In our efforts to avoid separating knowledge from meaning, experience, and practices, we will also talk only about 'disease' and not illness, since a multiplicity as both a patient's 'dis-ease' and a specific 'disease' is already built into this concept (Mol 2002).

The following excerpt is taken from a consultation between a male doctor (50) and a female patient (58) who recently returned from a trip to East Asia with an acting class she teaches. She started feeling ill and initially thought it was due to the polluted air: After having explained the course of her condition, the patient suddenly proclaims in a tone which could be either serious or ironic: 'Naturally, I think I must have contracted swine flu, bird flu or Ebola'. The doctor laughs lightly, and she continues: 'I just want you to tell me, "You are healthy, you can go home"; or that you give me some penicillin because I'm not feeling well'. Although there is quite an amount of dramatic staging of fear of exotic diseases in this excerpt, such interaction is rather typical of our data, as well as data from other studies (e.g. Stivers 2007). The patient seeks medical consultation due to an experience of dis-ease. She feels sick, and she is worried about what it might be.

Drawing on what might be termed a Western rationalist bio-medical logic of health and disease, she expects the GP to be able to resolve her state of dis-ease by way of producing 'objective' knowledge on aetiological origins as the foundation for positive treatment recommendations. But here, as in many other cases throughout our observations, dis-ease is not always so easily objectified as disease and pinpointed to a simple, specific origin. This lack of a clear diagnosis prevents the patient's experience of dis-ease from being promptly treated.

10.4.1 Liminal Zones of Uncertainty

In our attempt to explain how this neglected but fundamental aspect of medical practice can lead to over-prescription of antibiotics, we draw on the concept of 'liminal zones' as introduced by Stenner and Moreno-Gabriel (2013) drawing on the work of Victor Turner (1995). Liminal zones emerge when subjects are in a transition stage, entailing a condition of being on the edge of becoming something/someone else. The liminal is the phase of being 'betwixt and between' positions. The liminal phase often involves being in a condition of high arousal or intensity, since one—in this case—is neither sick nor healthy. Instead one is stuck in the middle, between these two states or positions, which entails both uncertainty and ensuing worries. When a patient's dis-ease is translated into disease and an antibiotic is prescribed, such a liminal zone is rapidly passed. The patient 'becomes' someone who is actually 'sick'. Her visit is legitimized, and she is reassured because her condition is now knowable and therefore often also treatable.

A consequence of analysing clinical encounters from such a perspective is that it becomes necessary to broaden our understanding of what biomedical knowledge and diagnostic categories such as 'bacterial pharyngitis' actually *do* in practice. Deploying the terminology of Greco (2017), a diagnosis works as a 'good' explanation in the sense that it both reassures the patient and legitimates the visit to the doctor. Hence, explanations and diagnoses must be understood as more than just 'more or less accurate representations of the patient's condition, but as efficacious interventions with therapeutic and social value in their own right' (p. 13). Turning to the pragmatic value of explanations, instead of interrogating their claim to a scientific 'truth', Greco demonstrates how explanations 'work' because they (a) acknowledge and validate the patient's sense of suffering without dismissing the reality and significance of symptoms, (b) provide 'tangible mechanisms' for explaining symptoms with the patient as 'active interlocutor', and (c) offer the possibility of connecting physical symptoms with psychosocial dimensions.

If we return to the above-mentioned doctor-patient encounter, it becomes easier to understand the pragmatic value of using (bio-)medical explanations even when no clear diagnosis or positive treatment recommendation is possible:

The doctor begins to examine her, listening to her breath with a stethoscope to her back while she is coughing and groaning heavily. He then asks the patient to follow him into the room next to the consultation room so that he can take a blood sample in order to do a CRP-test; this test will determine whether her condition is caused by a virus or bacteria. After having received the results of the CRP, the doctor states: 'Well, you do have an infection. You certainly do. But it is most likely due to a virus'. The patient responds: 'What does that mean? That it will pass with time?' The doctor explains that this is probably the case, but that she should contact the medical helpline if it gets any worse. At this point, the doctor is interrupted by the patient, who exclaims in a harsh voice: 'Hey—now I'm getting confused! You went inside my body', pointing to the spot where she was pricked by the needle, 'and we went into that room, but you still cannot put it bluntly if it is "Yes" or "No"?'.

Even though the patient's skin has been pierced and blood removed from her veins for it to be translated into a numerical value, quantifying and objectifying her sense of being sick, it do not yield the certainty, reassurance, and legitimation of a knowable disease. This is to some extent expected from the culturally predominant logic about a medical consultation as a knowledge-practice.

She has an infection, but not much can be said with absolute certainty. In our terminology, what is lacking is a 'good explanation', coming forth as a 'will to knowledge' that is clearly frustrated when the GP is not capable of translating, or objectifying, the patients' experience of dis-ease 'in-there' to specific knowable disease 'out-here'. This leaves her lingering in the zone of liminal uncertainty, in between certified sickness and health with discomfort. She is still at risk of something even worse, and this raises the stakes and intensity, affect, and unease of the situation. And contrary to what one might assume, this example suggests that patients are not only or not even primarily concerned with a 'will to knowledge' in order to obtain treatment. In our Foucauldian reading, the patients' 'will to knowledge' is will to obtain knowledge as a means for regulating her affective states and having her worries and concerns redressed. We argue that for those consultations where no clear-cut knowledge or treatment recommendation can be given, it is of crucial importance to understand how GPs handle these liminal zones of uncertainty.

In the following sections, we analyse what we understand as prototypical strategies that GPs deploy in order to manage the uncertainty and affective states of these liminal zones without resorting to *knowledge* or prescription of antibiotics. We will attempt to show that these strategies—which we collect under the label of 'psy-medical competence'—are to be considered both crucial to and inseparable from medical practice.

10.4.2 Governing the Future Through the Present

As illustrated above, clear-cut diagnoses and simple origins are not always so easily produced. Values above a certain threshold are often taken at face value, as seemingly neutral and objective facts about the 'true' disease of patients. However, values that lie too close to this threshold or below pose serious challenges to the immediate trust in the numbers that our medical instruments evoke (Mol 2008). This reveals how numbers are not direct representations, providing us with binary yes/no-answers, but abstractions that must be interpreted within a context and in relation to a specific patient. As indicators, numbers make sense in relation to a prognosis, not a diagnosis, and they consist of a form that is configured as probabilities rather than certainties. To decide and act against the background of probabilities is commonplace practice within medical care, but when numbers do not bring the relief that the trust in their objectivity implies, the intensity of the liminal zone of uncertainty intensifies, voices are raised, fingers pointed, and emotions stirred. Within the example, the GP tries to move the patient into another form of knowledge, the calculus of probabilities, in the following way:

> The GP runs through a range of options in relation to the various scenarios: it is most likely that the patient has come down with a virus infection, but if she does not feel better within 24 hours, she should go to the pharmacy and pick up a prescription, which he will put up on the server. If her condition has not improved over the weekend, she should contact the medical emergency to obtain something stronger. Furthermore, he schedules a follow-up consultation three weeks later in order to listen to

her lungs and make sure that she is feeling better. The patient summarizes: 'Okay, I just need to make sure that I have understood you correctly' after which she repeats the three different scenarios that the GP just listed and what she should do in each case.

Drawing on a Foucauldian understanding of risk, as outlined in the introductory chapter, one could term the GP's behaviour a kind of anticipatory 'risk management' strategy, since probabilities concerning dangers and difficulties are calculated, balanced, and dispersed in order to identify possible threats and weigh up the options of the present in relation to calculated future(s). As such, risk management involves a certain kind of calculative rationality aimed at ordering the present, rendering it understandable and governable, by locating it in a possible temporal trajectory with definite, but to some extent unpredictable, outcomes (Dean 1999). However, such strategies necessarily entail drawbacks and adverse effects. First of all, the materialization of risks within the present is not just a means to ensure oneself and others against possible threats in the future. It also raises the awareness of the uncontrollability of these threats. The way human beings relate to the risks represented by a calculative rationality is hardly ever as rational and uni-dimensional as the rationality itself (Lupton 2013). This means that moving from a strategy of certainties to one of probabilities, aiming at a prognosis rather than a diagnosis must imply an attention to its relation to the level of (perceived) uncertainty within the liminal zone at stake.

After having turned to the rationality of probabilities, the GP introduces another inter-related way of managing liminal zones of uncertainty, we term this *governing the present through the future*. The GP runs through a range of options in relation to various scenarios, still following a logic belonging to the realm of probabilities, transferring the experience of this realm on to the patient, who then summarizes the options. In the sequence above, it therefore becomes clear how the GP governs the liminal zone of uncertainty precisely by leaving it uncertain, by not giving in to any expectations (either his own or those of the patient) that her illness has some definitive diagnosis. Instead, the GP taps into and modulates the patient's experience of risk as well as her affective states by invoking various options into the present, creating what GPs call a 'safety-net'. In this way, he governs the liminal zone of uncertainty through an imaginary whereby future mechanisms of control temporarily prolong the present state of unease and reduces the perceived urgency for knowledge through the proposing of several potential treatment recommendations, all of which extend the care that he provides into the future.

10.4.3 Humouring the Steam Out of Persisting Worries

After having summarized the possible courses of action, the patient nevertheless returns to her initial worries:

> And the chance that I am suffering from Ebola?' the patient asks. The GP starts laughing and proclaims: 'I can with one hundred per cent certainty tell you that you are not suffering from Ebola. And I can with one hundred per cent certainty say that you are not suffering from bird flu or swine flu. And I can with one hundred per cent say, that you are not suffering from plague or cholera either', which makes both parts burst into laughter.

For an outsider, the commentaries above could seem a bit extreme. Does the patient seriously consider the possibility that she could be suffering from Ebola? Is she really taking this to be a risk? Is she merely adapting a persona for the stage? Or is she just joking? Is the GP actually making fun of his patient? And is it ever really a good idea to make light of such serious matters? In order to make sense of this, we focus on the complex ways in which psychological, affective, and cultural processes are intertwined in the clinical encounter and how the GP deploys strategies emanating from a psy-medical competence to handle these multifaceted relations.

If we start once more with *the patient*, we need to consider how experiences are always culturally mediated. Massumi (1993) argues that individuals in societies governed to a large extent by a rationality of risk are subjected to a constant 'low-level fear. A kind of background radiation saturating existence' (p. 24). Today, dangers are ubiquitous: second-hand smoke, parabens and radiance; multidrug resistant bacteria and mutated viruses, terrorism and climate change. Massumi argues that these hazards are managed by the individual through a continuous alertness to risks—

both the probable risks and those that are highly unlikely—in relation to which she/he produces and manages seemingly rational choices through self-regulation. If we follow this argument and spell out some possible consequences for the ways in which individuals monitor and regulate their health, Greco (1993) argues that in contemporary societies, refusal to properly consider or avoid possible threats 'is considered a failure of the self to take care of itself—a form of irrationality, or simply a lack of skilfulness' (p. 31). According to such a governmentality perspective, we should not judge the patient's way of relating to and handling risk with regard to how these actions and attitudes correlate with a medical logic of calculated probabilities. On the contrary, what is at stake is how to obtain knowledge and use this to skilfully maintain the balance between too much and too little concern for our health. This is a delicate balance, since we are constantly subjected to the task of judging our culturally mediated bodily (affective) experiences in relation to discourses of risk and in relation to the ever-changing criteria for being recognized as reasonable citizens. If we return to the above-mentioned consultation, the patient is to all appearances both exaggerating and dramatizing her fears about her current state. This staging actually allows her to verbalize and express her feelings of being in a state of unknown dis-ease, of being betwixt-and-between sickness and health, keeping open the possibility that she has more serious diseases without compromising her status as a reasonable subject.

Against this background, the response of the GP now stands out as a form of skilful 'double-communication'. He does not brush aside the worries of the patient as non-rational behaviour. Instead, he tries to manage this liminal zone of uncertainty by attending to her worries while concurrently defusing the affective investment in these worries.

Initially, he laughs a bit at the worries that she has voiced, but he then goes on to examine her. After the examination, where no clear-cut diagnosis or prescription can be given, his attention is led back to her worries, which have not been calmed since she is still suspended in liminality. He listens attentively, recognizing her as both a reasonable and rational subject, and as he dismisses the idea that this could be something serious, he also laughs. When asked in the following interview, he explains that his handling of the patient was related to the humorous way in which she presented herself, so it is 'not totally real'. At the same time, he recognizes that 'of course she has had some thoughts about it'. Hence, instead of dismissing her out of hand, he considers her anxieties as important in their own right:

> GP: [W]e want to terminate the consultation without there being any unnecessary worries when the patient leaves the room. It is not always possible, but with the means we have at hand, I think it must be considered reasonable that we do the things that are needed if the patient is to leave without unnecessary worries and thoughts. That can be troublesome in itself.

Nevertheless, the way the patient's anxieties are dealt with needs to be modified in proportion to the actual probability of the risks in question. As the GP explains, he would not have chosen to throw in the remark about plague and cholera unless he was convinced that the patient herself was aware that her experiences were 'sort of nuts'. At a communicative level, he then both accepts and responds to her questions, positioning her as an 'active interlocutor'. She is viewed as rational enough to pose relevant questions, but simultaneously extending her partial irony to a point where she indicates some real anxiety. The GP deploys his medical knowledge so as to diffuse her anxiety, placing her worries outside the rational discourse through his jokes, bringing down the level of liminal affectivity, even though no diagnosis is given nor any antibiotics prescribed. The consultation is thus an example of how psy-medical competence is used. We observe how medical knowledge combines with the ability to attend to understand and empathize with the patient, thus making for a flexible response. Moreover, we observe how communication, timing and the deployment of various affective strategies are intertwined in a way that recognizes and produces the patient as a legitimate and reasonable subject, managing the patient's affective states without making her feel ridiculed or ignored.

10.5 Conclusion

In the efforts to combat antibiotic resistance and over-prescription, there has been a preoccupation with acting, thinking, and governing through *knowledge* in accordance with a bio-medical logic.

As we have tried to demonstrate, this approach needs to be accompanied by more integrative and transdisciplinary approaches. Our approach has been one of affirmative critique, deploying different theories and approaches to broaden our understanding of what actually goes on in clinical consultations.

Introducing the concept of 'liminal zone of uncertainty', we suggest that states of not-knowing, risk, uncertainty, and worry need to be considered and analysed as essential phenomena in clinical practice. We have sought to demonstrate how GPs make use of a wide range of different strategies in order to manage and govern these 'liminal zones of uncertainty' in ways that affect, disrupt, resist, or modulate the bio-medical logic and the ubiquitous will to knowledge.

In order to conceptualize the competencies involved in such processes, we have suggested the term 'psy-medical competence'. We propose that further investigation be undertaken into how GPs acquire and utilize psy-medical competencies. Here it should be noted that we consider psy-medical competence as something more specific than the broad concept of 'patient-centred medicine'. Psy-medical competence is dynamic as well as person- and context-related. The specific strategies we have discussed are therefore not to be understood as an exhaustive list, model, figure, or textbook standard that can be directly transferred from one GP to another, in any setting with any type of patient. Rather, we consider these strategies as prototypical, in the sense that they open up the possibility for a line of inquiry and a way of doing research that feeds into the processes of reflection and discussion among GPs as to which strategies can be deployed when governing liminal zones of uncertainty and the affect implied by these zones in their everyday professional practice. Our main finding is that strategies intended to counteract or resist the propensity to *know* in a bio-medical sense are fundamental in order to handle what is a primary task within general practice: to relieve patients of the emotional stress and excess anxiety related to their experience of dis-ease. Central to this task lies the need for such relief to be performed in a way that does not compromise the status of the patient as both a reasonable and legitimate user of health care services, but on the contrary support the patient's resources to manage their own cognitive, affective, and somatic experience with confidence, balancing their understanding of too much or too little risk and uncertainty.

In the short term, making use of such strategies to govern patients' liminal affectivity might lower the perceived pressure for biological explanations and medical solutions. This is particularlyrelevant for unnecessary antibiotic consumption, since it is already known that a large proportion of prescribed antibiotics within general practice is prescribed on an insufficient basis. Further research into the acts, thoughts, and affects arising within liminal zones of uncertainty could therefore be valuable for training GPs in how to handle the ubiquitous will to knowledge that patients, or 'customers', of today demand of their physicians.

In a long-term perspective, the discovery of antibiotics and the widespread will to knowledge within modern societies—despite its many positive impacts—has also resulted in a sort of 'fiction' that all dangers can be known and eliminated, that all diseases have a knowable cause and a particular treatment. With such a background, we believe that alternative strategies are essential, as these may be conducive to the 'production'—or subjectification—of patients who come to understand themselves not just in terms of a bio-medical logic when confronted with dis-ease, but as bio-psycho-social subjects. Presumably, this would lower the patients' 'demand' for objective facts and an exact diagnosis due to a greater tolerance towards the unknowable and/or unknown and the uncertainty implied in such a state. As a result, one could hope that this would produce citizens who are more reflective when relating to their selves, bodies, disease, and health; and it would stimulate professionals to consider their role within a broader framework than that of biomedically based diagnosis/treatment.

References

Ackerman, S. L., Gonzales, R., Stahl, M. S., & Metlay, J. P. (2013). One size does not fit all: Evaluating an intervention to reduce antibiotic prescribing for acute bronchitis. *BMC Health Services Research, 13*(1), 462.

Cordoba, G., Siersma, V., Lopez-Valcarcel, B., Bjerrum, L., Llor, C., Aabenhus, R., & Makela, M. (2015). Prescribing style and variation in antibiotic prescriptions for sore throat: Cross-sectional study across six countries. *BMC Family Practice, 16*, 7.

Dean, M. (1999). Risk, calculable and incalculable. *Risk and Sociological Theory: New Directions and Perspectives, 1*(1998), 131–159.

Duane, S., Domegan, C., Callan, A., Galvin, S., Cormican, M., Bennett, K., … Vellinga, A. (2016). Using qualitative insights to change practice: Exploring the culture of antibiotic prescribing and consumption for urinary tract infections. *BMJ Open, 6*(1), e008894.

Gonzalez-Gonzalez, C., López-Vázquez, P., Vázquez-Lago, J. M., Piñeiro-Lamas, M., Herdeiro, M. T., Arzamendi, P. C., & Figueiras, A. (2015). Effect of physicians' attitudes and knowledge on the quality of antibiotic prescription: A cohort study. *PLoS ONE, 10(10)*, 1–12.

Greco, M. (1993). Psychosomatic subjects and the duty to be well: Personal agency within medical rationality. *Economy and Society, 3*(22), 357–372.

Greco, M. (2017). Pragmatics of explanation: Creative accountability in the care of 'medically unexplained symptoms'. *The Sociological Review, 65*(2_Suppl), 110–129. https://doi.org/10.1177/0081176917710425

Grol, R., Wensing, M., Eccles, M., & Davis, D. (Eds.). (2013). *Improving patient care: The implementation of change in health care* (2nd ed.). West Sussex: John Wiley & Sons.

Hansen, M. P., Hoffmann, T. C., McCullough, A. R., van Driel, M. L., & Del Mar, C. B. (2015, February). Antibiotic resistance: What are the opportunities for primary care in alleviating the crisis? *Front Public Health, 3*(February), 35.

Jakobsen, K. A., Melbye, H., Kelly, M. J., Ceynowa, C., Mölstad, S., Hood, K., & Butler, C. C. (2010). Influence of CRP testing and clinical findings on antibiotic prescribing in adults presenting with acute cough in primary care. *Scandinavian Journal of Primary Health Care, 28*(4), 229–236.

Jansbøl, K., Nielsen, A., Henriette, M., Jessica, M., Pia, L., & Kjellberg, K. (2012). *Hvordan påvirker kliniske vejledninger almen praksis? Hvordan har kliniske vejledninger ændret almen praksis?* (pp. 237–750). Månedsskrift for almen praksis, September 2012.

Jørgensen, L. C., Friis Christensen, S., Cordoba Currea, G., Llor, C., & Bjerrum, L. (2013). Antibiotic prescribing in patients with acute rhinosinusitis is not in agreement with European recommendations. *Scandinavian Journal of Primary Health Care, 31*(2), 101–105.

Lopez-Vazquez, P., Vazquez-Lago, J. M., & Figueiras, A. (2012). Misprescription of antibiotics in primary care: A critical systematic review of its determinants. *Journal of Evaluation in Clinical Practice, 18*, 473–484.

Lupton, D. (2013). *Risk* (2nd ed.). London: Routledge.

Massumi, B. (1993). *The politics of everyday fear*. Minneapolis: University of Minnesota Press.

Mol, A. (2002). *The body multiple: Ontology in medical practice*. Durham and London: Duke University Press.

Mol, A. (2008). *The logic of care: Health and the problem of patient choice*. Oxon and New York: Routledge.

Rodrigues, A. T., Ferreira, M., Roque, F., Falcão, A., Ramalheira, E., Figueiras, A., & Herdeiro, M. T. (2016). Physicians' attitudes and knowledge concerning antibiotic prescription and resistance: Questionnaire development and reliability. *BMC Infectious Diseases, 16*(1), 7.

Stenner, P., & Moreno-Gabriel, E. (2013). Liminality and affectivity: The case of deceased organ donation. *Subjectivity, 6*(3), 229–253.

Stivers, T. (2007). *Prescribing under pressure: Parent-physician conversations and antibiotics*. Oxford: Oxford University Press.

Strandberg, E. L., Brorsson, A., Hagstam, C., Troein, M., & Hedin, K. (2013). "I'm Dr Jekyll and Mr Hyde": Are GPs' antibiotic prescribing patterns contextually dependent? A qualitative focus group study. *Scandinavian Journal of Primary Health Care, 31*(3), 158–165.

Timmermans, S., & Berg, M. (2003). *The gold standard: The challenge of evidence-based medicine and standardization in health care*. Philadelphia: Temple University Press.

Tonkin-Crine, S., Walker, A. S., & Butler, C. C. (2015, June). Contribution of behavioural science to antibiotic stewardship. *BMJ, 350*(June), h3413.

Turner, V. (1995). *The ritual process: Structure and anti-structure*. Piscataway, NJ: Transaction Publishers.

11

The Antibiotic Challenge: Justifications for Antibiotic Usage in the World of Medicine

Kim Sune Jepsen and Inge Kryger Pedersen

11.1 Introduction: The Antibiotic Challenge from a Sociological Perspective

In our era of a risk society (Beck 1992), risking resistance to antibiotics has become a scientific, social, and political problem. The excessive and inappropriate usage of antibiotics to cure diseases within the human and veterinary sectors has led to increasing resistance among bacteria (such as Methicillin-resistant *Staphylococcus aureus*, MRSA), which poses a risk to human health and society. This indeterminate situation raises unresolved political questions about how best to avoid the unsustainable route to a potential global problem from resistant bacteria that easily transcend national borders (e.g. through the import of food products, migration,

K. S. Jepsen (✉)
Department of Sociology, Lund University, Lund, Sweden
e-mail: kim.jepsen@outlook.com

I. K. Pedersen
Department of Sociology, University of Copenhagen, Copenhagen, Denmark
e-mail: ikp@soc.ku.dk

C. S. Jensen et al. (eds.), *Risking Antimicrobial Resistance*,
https://doi.org/10.1007/978-3-319-90656-0_11

tourism, etc.), thus making efforts at governance difficult on a national basis alone. With a lack of new therapeutic agents in the pharmaceutical pipelines (ECDC 2009), there is accordingly a strong national and international political 'push' to restrict antibiotic usage so as to avoid 'the antibiotic paradox' of a cure that leads to resistance (Levy 2002). This push entails comprehensive national and international surveillance programmes such as those from the European Centre for Disease Prevention and Control (ECDC 2013), as well as recommendations for the need to change professional expert practices to accommodate more prudent usage, better diagnostics, restrictive guidelines, more efficient control mechanisms based on laboratory studies, and the optimizing of national and international surveillance programmes (WHO 2001, p. 4; 2012).

Although professionals such as microbiologists now speak of a 'post-antibiotic apocalypse' in which centuries of modern medicine and its advanced forms of treatments are jeopardized by the lack of antibiotic cures (Nerlich and James 2009), the less dramatic formulation of current policy encompasses a call for changing usage and generating new innovations in the field of science, expertise, and technologies within a 'One Health' perspective. 'One Health' aims to develop new antibiotics and to support scientific, political, and technological interventions to take into account intersectional problems of resistant bacterial tribes in a holistic manner (EC 2012, p. 4). This entails a call for more thorough examinations of current antibiotic applications and more prudent and rational usage across divisions of societal sectors and species. The need for increased scrutiny applies also to the Nordic countries, including Denmark, which are among the least-infected European countries with comprehensive surveillance and administrative policies in place. Now the experience of increasing resistance is leading to the implementation of new international and national policy standards and measures of innovation, surveillance, and restrictions (DANMAP 2014).

In this chapter, we respond to the call for more thorough explorations of current antibiotic applications in society, thus looking more closely at the reasons and moral concerns underlying medical experts' antibiotic usage in clinical practices. Similar to other scholars of sociology and science studies (e.g. Beck 1992; 1996), we are concerned with exploring how uncertain *socio-natural issues* (in our case, antibiotic usage and resistance) come to matter in society through the ways that science and expertise frame and intervene in the difficulties of 'handling natural problems'. As many studies have demonstrated by exploring expert cultures of science, along with how expertise operates in practice, scientific interventions are regularly based on cultural commitments, values, and norms, which orient scientific work but often remain unacknowledged. Such ignorance of the social or cultural dimension may subsequently lead to unrealistic understandings that complex socio-natural problems can be solved with a scientific 'fix' outside more general discussions of what kind of social consequences may unintentionally follow and the inherently risky uncertainties (Beck 1992, p. 81; Jasanoff 2004; Wynne 2002). Accordingly, we explore the reasons, cultural commitments, and reflexive strategies that orientate current antibiotic usage within a particular expert culture of general practitioners (GPs) and their clinical treatment practices and strategies.

The main contribution of this chapter is to provide a micro-sociological perspective on a particular expert culture and its concerns in facing the antibiotic challenge. This turns out to be far from a simple matter of applying antibiotics to cure diseases. Instead, our explorations find that medical experts, when deciding whether or not to prescribe, adopt different reflexive strategies and exhibit varying moral concerns about what constitutes the common good. Thus, it is hoped the focus on the complex concerns of actual professions might provide a basis for understanding the genuine social complexities of antibiotic usage by experts and how such usage originates in practical reasons and concerns, all of which need to be taken into account when crafting future policies to control the antibiotic challenge. Hence, the question we pursue, explore, and elaborate on in this chapter is the following: By what means do medical professionals practising within a certain expert culture justify the usage of antibiotics? Drawing on French pragmatism and its regime model of justification (Boltanski and Thévenot 2006), we demonstrate GPs' moral and social concerns, discussing how antibiotic usage (or not) can be understood as a matter of how GPs pursue and justify different treatment strategies.

11.2 The Model of Justification: The Social Logic of Settling Indeterminate Situations

Relatively few sociological investigations have explored the antibiotic challenge and its impact on contemporary modern societies. Current sociological analyses have explored especially the social representations of antibiotic resistance in UK media. Such analyses have helped to reveal how we talk about and understand the antibiotic problem in terms of an emerging catastrophe discourse in microbiology (Nerlich and James 2009), as a disruption of social and moral order in public institutions (Washer and Joffe 2006), and as new obligations to self-monitor as a means of complying with an era of neoliberal governance and a moral emphasis on individual responsibilities (Brown and Crawford 2009, p. 520). In distinction, and following the call of the 'One Health perspective', we are concerned with how expert cultures engage with antibiotic usage and resistance, and how such practices are qualified and justified. In order to pursue this issue, we look more closely at clinical practice through a sociological theory and model developed to account for how people in general *can* resolve indeterminate situations in daily life by recourse to different principles and modes of justification.

The guiding question of the renowned theory outlined in *On Justification* (Boltanski and Thévenot 2006) is how people manage to subject their situational circumstances to reflexive scrutiny and normative evaluations in order to settle and reach agreements in practical matters and controversial affairs. The pragmatic proposition is that situations of uncertainty or disagreement are common in everyday life and that people often need to justify their actions in accordance with general principles of what is right (Ibid., p. 32). That is, situations in which order disintegrates, uncertainties are high, or disagreements occur make it necessary for actors to reflexively resort to critical interrogations: What matters? Is this fair? What principles should count? Who and what should be included in the assessed situation and the actions that are involved in order to come to a good solution? Such issues make up the normative action of testing and associating how things matter in respect to indeterminate everyday life situations. The reflexive moral act of justification is understood as the act of moving beyond personal idiosyncrasies towards the provision of general arguments in view of what is deemed right and in the interest of the common good in a given situation (Boltanski and Thévenot 2000).

Exploring ordinary indeterminate situations, Boltanski and Thévenot have constructed an elaborate theoretical and methodological model for capturing the moral grammars of people's ordinary evaluative actions. The model of justification is grounded and qualified by drawing on six classical political philosophies,[1] thus providing an analytical perspective on how certain conventional orders or regimes support and constrain actions in respect to different rationalities, principles of worth, and notions of the common good. Hence, a common denominator of political philosophies is that they seek to establish principles of equivalence between people and things in respect to a notion of the common good for humanity. The sociological suggestion, however, is that within modern complex societies there exists a plurality of different conventional orders to which people refer as a means of justifying and settling indeterminate or conflictual situations. That is, social actions take place within more or less institutionalized social worlds—regimes—that both constrain and provide support for people's critical and reflexive capacities in terms of shared competences to evaluate situations (Ibid., p. 66). On this account, the model constructs and operates with different regimes of justification that embody distinct higher principles of worth for justifying actions (Boltanski and Thévenot 2006, pp. 170–200).

In the *inspirational regime*, worth rests on a principle of particular grace or sainthood with judgements based on passion, emotional attachments, and creativity (e.g. the inspired artist); the common good is represented by the uniqueness and originality of the particular person who speaks for all. In the *domestic regime*, worth is based on hierarchical positions and personalized relations of trust, which generate authority and esteem; tradition is of crucial importance (e.g. the elder), and the common good consists in establishing a tradition of respect, responsibilities,

[1] The philosophies of the different conventional orders are Augustine's 'order of inspiration', Bossuet's 'domestic order', Hobbes' 'order of fame', Rousseau's 'civic order', Smith's 'market', and Saint-Simon's 'industrial order'.

and personal bonds of trust. In the *regime of fame*, worth is based purely on the opinion and esteem of others supported by the importance of signs that generate respect (e.g. the famous actor); the common good is a social bond secured by recognition. In the *civic regime*, worth is attached to the one who expresses or embodies the general will and manages to take on a symbolic role to benefit civic life (e.g. the politician); the common good lies in the capacity of representing others as members of a collective—in a civic authority who expresses people's common aspiration. In the *market regime*, worth is based on making a fortune by offering goods in a competitive marketplace and being able to seize the right opportunities (e.g. businessperson); the common good is the possession of common objects that others desire and that secures social attachments. Finally, in the *industrial regime*, worth is based on performance, instrumental planning, efficiency, and productivity (e.g. the expert); the common good is control and responsibility over actions that secure normal stability and progress for all.

A foundational element of the model is how the ascription of worth to people, things, and objects in social situations takes place by testing arrangements in accord with the aforementioned principles: 'When they are used for critique and justification in public arenas, these orders face a 'reality test' involving the material environment' (Thévenot 2009, p. 798). A reality test is the application of principles and moral grammars that are used to sort out uncertain situations by evaluating how objects and things matter to the public, that is, what is worth taking into account and how to justify such matters vis-à-vis the common good. A reality test basically entails mobilizing qualified justifications of how uncertain situations matter, that is, it demonstrates a proof or principle of how circumstances have implications for the common good (Boltanski 2012, p. 45).

This model of plural justificatory regimes has been further developed to include a 'green order of worth' that directly addresses sustainability, environmental friendliness and renewability (Thévenot et al. 2000, p. 241). The ecological worth concerns the preservation of entities in the environment as a common good: the manner in which farm sites are maintained, as well as efforts to promote clean air and biodiversity, can all be seen as issues related to a sustainable green order ranging from small natural entities to large phenomena. The green regime involves ecological justifications, that is, how nature and natural entities matter to society as a means of achieving the common good.

As we will demonstrate, the regime model for understanding the medical rationales of treatment strategies (as the situational object of study) opens the way for systematic empirical explorations of the significant reasons and moral concerns that support antibiotic usage within an expert culture. Furthermore, this approach also contributes to current public health studies of antibiotic usage, which indicate that social factors are significant to how diseases are understood and engaged with (Butler et al. 1998; Gjelstad et al. 2011; Høye et al. 2010; Kumar et al. 2003; Petursson 2005; Simpson et al. 2007). What such studies suggest is that clinical practitioners routinely need to incorporate flexible negotiations of a manifold of symptoms, individual life spans, and ad hoc negotiation of different situations, values, and ends. Although public health studies offer clear indications of the need to systematically explore the social concerns informing medical experts in their antibiotic treatment practices (for the Scandinavian context, see e.g. Høye et al. 2010; Llor and Bjerrum 2014), these studies do not seek to explain the moral framework and principles underlying medical work or to expose the social concerns that, in our view, may orient antibiotic treatments. As will be shown, the 'scientific reasons' for handling antibiotic usage can be seen to rely on multiple principles, social logic, and moral concerns linked to proper usage and what constitutes the common good.

11.3 The Plural Regimes of Antibiotic Justification in Clinical Practice

In taking such sociological steps to understand the clinical reasons for prescribing antibiotics, we look upon the clinic as a semi-public space in which issues of treatment and antibiotic usage are tested, qualified, and justified in regard to a general societal concern. Practitioners not only focus on how best to provide individual tailored care for citizens but also draw on other rationalities, principles, and standards for negotiating and justifying the application of antibiotics in respect to different situations and ends that go beyond the immediate care situation.

The empirical material consists of interviews with 21 Danish GPs. Semi-structured interviews were carried out to learn more about the GPs' practices and procedures for antibiotic treatment, including issues of respiratory tract infection, usage of national guidelines, professional collaboration, and physician views on the emerging problem of resistance (for more about methods and methodological considerations, see Pedersen and Jepsen 2018). The selection of these issues should be seen in light of the fact that 90 per cent of all antibiotics are prescribed in primary care in the human sector, and between 2004 and 2013, the overall consumption of broad-spectrum antimicrobial agents in humans increased by 72 per cent (DANMAP 2013, p. 15). Furthermore, recent evaluations of general practice in the Nordic countries have shown that respiratory tract infection is a leading reason for prescribing and that only 20 per cent of all prescriptions for infections are in fact medically appropriate (Llor Bjerrum 2014, p. 8). Let us now turn to the analysis of how different regimes of justification can be understood to support GPs' reflexive engagement with antibiotic usage in the medical clinic. We now present a selection of the regimes that we have found most significant in the empirical materials and as a means of understanding the clinical reasons and justifications voiced by GPs in public health care:

The industrial regime emphasizing the worth of planning, efficient strategies, and standardized test methods is a common pattern for securing good clinical treatments. On a given day, a doctor may consult between 20 and 30 patients, and efficiency and high performance is necessary to meet patients' specific needs. The industrial (paradigmatic) test serves as an extension of tools, protocol, and guidelines that function to support the act of evaluating a situation to ensure scientific proof and the common good of optimal functionality and normal operation (Boltanski and Thévenot 2006, p. 204, 210). From this perspective, a common justification of antibiotic usage is modelled on more or less standardized routines, codes, and guidelines, which support the rationale for tests, for example, blood samples and CRP (C-Reactive Protein Test). In the industrial regime, it is the interpretation of *standardized* examinations that is inscribed in test instruments and procedures, which in turn secures indicative knowledge of illnesses. As one doctor argued, the usage of guidelines in 'lægehåndbogen' (a general and common manual of diagnoses for medical professionals) was an important and efficient instrument: '...for me it's important to use the same guidelines all the time, because they're fastest, and because they get updated, they're written by skilled people...' (GP9).

An interesting example of standardizing treatment was how a senior doctor had developed an approach whereby nurses ran minor tests before the actual consultation, thus making it possible to have relatively objective indications to examining the patient: '...it began ten or twelve years ago, because we were very busy and had a lot of patients, and it was a way of systematizing things, so that they wouldn't take up too much time in the consultation and so that it would be possible to decide what to do in one or the other situation' (GP17). Yet it is also clear that management of efficiencies in daily care is far from unproblematic. As a doctor explained, diagnostics rest on a complicated calculation of multiple results that inform professional judgements: '...when you prescribe or decide something, then it is the whole arena you operate in and this arena is more than the single elements in my opinion, so sometimes we have to prescribe anyway, let's say in case pneumonia is a risk' (GP4).

Considerations such as the patient's general health, symptoms, comorbidity, and personal history are part of generating knowledge foundations for making sound judgements to secure and control efficient strategies for antibiotic treatment. Blood samples and standardized tests were thus also a means of supporting clinical diagnostics: 'I use it when I'm in doubt... and when I have to convince a patient when I'm certain. Normally, I'm not in doubt about whether they need [antibiotics] or not' (GP1). Within the industrial regime, justifications and tests for appropriate antibiotic usage thus centred on how best to administer efficiencies in treatment on the basis of standardized medical equipment, drawing on accounts of patient history and striking balances between different social issues (see also Chap. 9 for an enquiry into social issues).

The civic regime concerns the representative power of an authority to make decisions in the general interest of civic life. The maintenance of jurisdictional boundaries composed of knowledge, codes, and criteria supports control within an arena of practice that is crucial for exercising the role of a spokesperson who possesses authority to speak for the general interest (Boltanski and Thévenot 2006, p. 186, 192). Related issues that arose within the clinic concerned the responsibility of holding a public office for the common good: 'We've been given a responsibility, namely, the right to prescribe pharmaceuticals…and we also have a responsibility, if it has consequences for society' (GP1). The role of GP was qualified as a professional duty that would also include general concerns for civic life, such as securing an awareness-raising dialogue with patients about the limitations of antibiotic usage, taking time to carry out proper examinations, and addressing the need to do away with professional misunderstandings: '…we have to say that the idea antibiotics do no harm and it's better to be safe, is wrong. And we have to let go of this and say, well it's perfectly right that on a clinical basis you may choose to ask: 'Is this relevant?' But there has to be a reason' (GP12).

A particularly important concern was voiced in regard to how improvements in professional care could be undertaken. Several doctors called for a consultative institution in which collected data on clinical patterns of usage would be distributed on a regular basis. One doctor also underlined a problem with how past practices of care were dismantled: 'The professional community that we benefit the most from, and this has been cut down, was in days gone by when a colleague operating as a general medical consultant would review our consumption of all kinds of pharmaceutical drugs, including antibiotics. Then we were compared with others in the municipalities. At that point they could say: 'You use more broad-spectrum penicillin than on average, why?" (GP1).

In addition, the particular role as custodian of the public good was also vividly exemplified by how several doctors were unanimously concerned about the manner in which antibiotic usage was linked to increasing societal pressures: 'You see, there are enormous numbers of people in Denmark who aren't well, although we might not think this is case, and so there's huge pressure for them to live up to the demands of the labour market and all kinds of other affairs….to walk around ill for three weeks or something because of a respiratory tract infection—there's no time for this. That is, you see people have a complete breakdown if you refuse them antibiotics for sinusitis, which is also a respiratory tract infection. For me it's self-evident. If the condition has lasted for more than three weeks, they'll simply get [antibiotics] or else they'll walk around with their problems for an enormously long time. On the other hand, one might say, yes, it will get better on its own, but this isn't how patients are prepared to live with it' (GP7). In this sense, the justifications and test for good antibiotic usage were tied to larger concerns about changing professional attitudes, taking into account general public health and societal pressures on patients′ general livelihood.

In the domestic regime, justifications are linked to personal ties along with attachments to the local, and the value of tradition and proximity are mobilized in the qualification of how situations matter. Proper antibiotic usage was qualified in terms of the local settings for clinical practice that would entail close and familiar contact with patients. The worth of familiar arrangements can be understood in distinction to the industrial regime of creating efficiencies based on planning, instruments, and standardization. As a younger doctor explained in relation to the value of CRP, 'We don't treat numbers, we treat patients, because I actually think that the clinical is more important than the numbers. Of course, one can use numbers for support when in doubt, at least once in a while anyway' (GP6). In this sense, domestic justifications mainly concerned how close contact and intimate clinical knowledge of particular patients would secure sound evaluations in matters of antibiotic care. As a senior doctor explained: 'We have very little technology at our disposal, and if we haven't got that, then we have to trust our clinical experience' (GP17).

If the domestic qualifications of treatment were linked to familiarity with patients—'a localized knowledge' tailored to the individual patient—then this was further qualified and nuanced as a matter of different experiences. As a younger doctor underlined: 'I think that as a young doctor you're almost ideological, I was about to say. We are indeed brought up with the problem of antibiotic resistance, and I believe that I'm very strict compared with my older colleagues (...) I always start with narrow-spectrum antibiotics' (GP6). Yet the generational issue was also qualified in terms of accumulated experience and distinctive professional capabilities to navigate complex histories of illness: 'I believe that as a younger doctor you're always a bit more idealistic, because you've learned through your studies that there has to be this and that before one treats with antibiotics. So, you come out as more of an idealist than you will be two years later, because by then you've seen that it's smart to avoid conflicts and to become good friends with the patient for the sake of the future, when they might be seriously ill, and then they'll come instead of having left angry' (GP3). While several doctors did therefore underline generational differences in prescription patterns, the basic qualifications and justifications centred on how familiarity with patients and localized knowledge can support good antibiotic usage.

The green environmental regime values the solidarity between means and ends, that is, not treating natural entities as a means but as an end itself (Latour 1998). Justifications place worth on the accountability for socio-natural consequences, and moral engagement is geared to protecting the collective environments of both humans and non-humans (Thévenot et al. 2000, p. 257). As one doctor argued, 'I think as a doctor you need to be aware that the problem with too much antibiotic consumption is the resistance that follows…we risk widespread resistance against antibiotics. If this happens, then modern medicine is finished. You won't be able to have ordinary surgical operations with antibiotics that reduce the infection and complication ratios…There are so many fundamental and basic scientific inventions that are based on antibiotics. So, the prospects for the future are unbelievably gloomy if we end up returning to a 'pre-antibiotic era', as they call it' (GP12). Green justifications above all concerned the manner in which resistance would be an unintended and uncontrollable risk to human health and society if consumption of antibiotics were not changed: 'It's so easy to give [antibiotics], but in return you heighten the risk of resistance. In regard to your question if resistance is a problem on the level of individual care, no, it isn't. It matters on the societal level' (GP9).

With respect to particular green issues, several doctors expressed worries about current usage within the veterinary sector when confronted with the question of significant challenges related to usage and resistance: 'The biggest challenge or worry is whether there will be interventions…. when you hear what farming is using, what's put in the food, sure I can try to cut down on antibiotic usage in some cases where it's borderline, and it's the small details that determine if it goes one way or the other [the decision to prescribe], if they're putting it in the food, though, then I sometimes wonder whether my restrictive guidelines and rules matter at all' (GP6).

In this sense, antibiotic usage and its relation to increasing resistance were qualified in ways that extended far beyond the clinic to issues of how other professional fields were operating and larger societal changes were needed. In particular, a recurrent qualification of how to ensure good prescription practice centred on its role as a common political problem that concerned many professional groups and ultimately had to be addressed at the level of policy and collective interventions. This was framed very concisely by a doctor: '...we might need to see this as a whole ecological problem, and not the responsibility of the medics or the human sector ... resistant genes are transferred from one bacteria to the other...there are some political decisions that must be made beyond what I decide in my consultations' (GP6).

11.4 Conclusion

The medical clinic can be seen as an arena in which the justification of antibiotic usage follows diverse modes of qualifying and justifying treatment strategies. As we have seen, the application of antibiotics is accompanied by different moral valuations and justifications concerned with efficiencies, general civic interests, localized knowledge, and more pervasive 'green issues' linked to how to secure sustainable societal usage through political intervention. In regard to clinical practice, one of the core medical challenges is to navigate different ends and to make informed and appropriate choices in specific situations where antibiotics might be prescribed. We might say that clinical practice navigates an area of tension in which antibiotic applications intersect with multiple forms of social logic, moral evaluations and justifications in the situated negotiation of when and why (not) to apply antibiotics. Such diverse moral dimensions within cultures of expertise need to be recognized and taken into account, and core stakeholders and their multiple concerns need to be brought to the table with the aim of crafting new policy interventions if we are to achieve consensus on how best to navigate the antibiotic challenge in the future.

If the model of justification has made it possible to explore how an expert culture of general practitioners qualifies, evaluates and justifies situations of antibiotic usage, we have left out an important aspect that deserves more research in future. Hence, an important insight of the regime model is that indeterminate situations are often comprised of, or arise between, different regimes, because people engage each other in critical controversies about finding right and fair solutions in uncertain situations. In this chapter, we have only touched upon such controversies, focusing more on providing insights into the different regimes or social worlds of qualifying and justifying what constitutes good antibiotic usage. However, this does not mean that critical controversies were not at all present. General practitioners, for instance, showed great concern about the standards of efficiency that underlie antibiotic usage in industrial farming and, according to some, lead to a breakdown of green sustainable usage as presented in the ecological regime. Yet, our approach and analysis also follow from the more dominant empirical patterns that emerged in the interviews. General practitioners reflexively navigate changing situations related to prescriptions with a deep-seated concern for what is good, reasonable, and justifiable practice, and the latter can be understood to follow different moral standards or principles of worth according to the regime in question. Rather than allowing themselves to become mired in controversial tensions, general practitioners demonstrate a capacity to shift between regimes and standards on qualified grounds, thus providing rich insights into the multiple justificatory logics of clinical expert practice.

References

Beck, U. (1992). *Risk society: Towards a new modernity*. London: Sage Publications.

Beck, U. (1996). World risk society as cosmopolitan society? Ecological questions in a framework of manufactured uncertainties. *Theory, Culture and Society, 13*(4), 1–32.

Boltanski, L. [1990] (2012). *Love and justice as competences*. Cambridge: Polity Press.

Boltanski, L., & Thévenot, L. (2000). The reality of moral expectations: A sociology of situated judgement. *Philosophical Explorations: An International Journal for the Philosophy of Mind and Action, 3*(3), 208–231.

Boltanski, L., & Thévenot, L. [1991] (2006). *On justification—Economies of worth*. Princeton, NJ: Princeton University Press.

Brown, B., & Crawford, P. (2009). 'Post antibiotic apocalypse': Discourses of mutation in narratives of MRSA. *Sociology of Health and Illness, 31*(4), 508–524.

Butler, C., Rollnick, S., Pill, R., Maggs-Rapport, F., & Stott, N. (1998). Understanding the culture of prescribing: Qualitative study of general practitioners' and patients' perceptions of antibiotics for sore throat. *British Medical Journal, 317*(7159), 637–642.

DANMAP. (2013). *DANMAP 2013—Use of antimicrobial agents and occurrence of antimicrobial resistance in bacteria from food animals, food and humans in Denmark*. The Danish Integrated Antimicrobial Resistance Monitoring and Research Program. Copenhagen: Statens Serum Institute, National Veterinary Institute, Technical University of Denmark, National Food Institute, Technical University of Denmark.

DANMAP. (2014). *Use of antimicrobial agents and occurrence of antimicrobial resistance in bacteria from food animals, food and humans in Denmark*. The Danish Integrated Antimicrobial Resistance Monitoring and Research Program. Copenhagen: Statens Serum Institute, National Veterinary Institute, Technical University of Denmark, National Food Institute, Technical University of Denmark.

EC. (2012). *Council conclusions on the impact of antimicrobial resistance in the human health sector and in the veterinary sector—A "One Health" perspective*. Brussels: The Council of the European Union.

ECDC. (2009). *The bacterial challenge: Time to react. A call to narrow the gap between multidrug-resistant bacteria in the EU and the development of new antibacterial agents*. European Centre for Disease Prevention and Control. Technical Report. Stockholm: ECDC.

ECDC. (2013). *Antimicrobial resistance surveillance in Europe*. Annual report of the European Antimicrobial Resistance Surveillance Network (EARS-Net). European Centre for Disease Prevention and Control. Stockholm: ECDC.

Gjelstad, S., Straand, J., Dalen, I., Fetveit, A., Strom, H., & Lindbaek, M. (2011). Do general practitioners' consultation rates influence their prescribing patterns of antibiotics for acute respiratory tract infections? *Journal of Antimicrobial Chemotherapy, 66*(10), 2425–2433.

Høye, S., Frich, J., & Lindbæk, M. (2010). Delayed prescribing for upper: Respiratory tract infections: A qualitative study of GPs' views and experience. *British Journal of General Practice, 60*(581), 907–912.

Jasanoff, S. (Ed.). (2004). *States of knowledges—The co-production of science and social order*. London: Routledge.

Kumar, S., Little, P., & Britten, N. (2003). Why do general practitioners prescribe antibiotics for sore throat? Grounded theory interview study. *British Medical Journal, 326*, 1–6.

Latour, B. (1998). To modernize or to ecologize? That's the question. In N. Castree & B. Willems-Braun (Eds.), *Remaking reality: Nature at the millenium* (pp. 221–242). London: Routledge.

Levy, S. (2002). *The antibiotic paradox: How the misuse of antibiotics destroy their curative power*. Cambridge: Perseus Publishing.

Llor, C., & Bjerrum, L. (2014). Antimicrobial resistance: Risk associated with antibiotic overuse and initiatives to reduce the problem. *Therapeutic Advances in Drug Safety, 5*(6), 229–241.

Nerlich, B., & James, R. (2009). "The post-antibiotic apocalypse" and the "war on superbugs": Catastrophe discourse in microbiology, its rhetorical form and political function. *Public Understanding of Science, 18*(5), 574–590.

Pedersen, I. K., & Jepsen, K. S. (2018). Prescribing antibiotics: General practitioners dealing with "non-medical issues"? *Professions & Professionalism, 8*(1) pp. 1–14

Petursson, P. (2005). GPs' reasons for "non-pharmacological" prescribing of antibiotics. *Scandinavian Journal of Primary Health Care, 23*, 120–125.

Simpson, S., Wood, F., & Butler, C. (2007). General practitioners' perceptions of antimicrobial resistance: A qualitative study. *Journal of Antimicrobial Chemotherapy, 59*, 292–296.

Thévenot, L. (2009). Postscript to the special issue: Governing life by standards—A view from engagements. *Social Studies of Science, 39*(5), 793–813.

Thévenot, L., Moody, M., & Lafaye, C. (2000). Forms of valuing nature: Arguments and modes of justification in French and American environmental disputes. In M. Lamont & L. Thévenot (Eds.), *Rethinking comparative cultural sociology: Repertoires of evaluation in France and the United States*. Cambridge: Cambridge University Press.

Washer, P., & Joffe, H. (2006). The "hospital superbug": Social representations of MRSA. *Social Science & Medicine, 63*(8), 2141–2152.

WHO. (2001). WHO global strategy for the containment of antimicrobial resistance. World Health Organization, WHO/CDS/CSR/DRS.2001.2.

Wynne, B. (2002). Risk and environment as legitimatory discourses of technology: Reflexivity inside out? *Current Sociology, 50*(3), 459–477.

12

Concluding Remarks on 'Risking Antimicrobial Resistance'

Carsten Strøby Jensen, Søren Beck Nielsen, and Lars Fynbo

12.1 Introduction

Over the last five years, there have been remarkable developments in the scope and nature of the policy initiatives that focus on combatting the spread of antimicrobial resistance (AMR) globally. The United Nations (UN), World Health Organization (WHO), Food and Agriculture Organization (FAO), European Union (EU), and Group of Seven (G7)

C. S. Jensen (✉)
Department of Sociology, University of Copenhagen, Copenhagen, Denmark
e-mail: csj@soc.ku.dk

S. B. Nielsen
Department of Nordic Studies and Linguistics, University of Copenhagen, Copenhagen, Denmark
e-mail: sbnielsen@hum.ku.dk

L. Fynbo
VIVE – The Danish Center for Social Science Research, Copenhagen, Denmark
e-mail: lafy@vive.dk

C. S. Jensen et al. (eds.), *Risking Antimicrobial Resistance*,
https://doi.org/10.1007/978-3-319-90656-0_12

are among the international organizations that have taken initiatives to develop strategies to combat AMR. The question remains, of course, as to whether the initiatives have been taken early enough to address the threats that project up to ten million people dying annually in the year 2050 as a result of AMR (O'Neill 2014).

International initiatives have been taken because the spread of AMR is viewed as a global problem. In part, the AMR population affects all regions and countries. Moreover, AMR threat does not stop at national borders. AMR is boundless, moving relatively effortlessly across borders, regions, and countries.

The international policy initiatives focus largely on restricting the use of antimicrobials. As is known, it is the use of antimicrobials that causes resistance and leads to AMR. The main objective of international policy initiatives, therefore, is to limit the spread of AMR through limiting the use of antimicrobials. 'Prudent use of antimicrobials' is one of the tools that have been developed in order to combat AMR. A very large proportion of the antibiotics used globally is used in situations where their effect is in fact very limited. It is estimated that up to 50 percent of the antimicrobials consumed by humans has no discernible health effect. For example, the infections may be carried by a virus and not by a bacterium, making the antimicrobial useless. Antimicrobials have effects only on those infections that are bacteria-borne and not on the infections that are virus-borne. One of the ways in which the consumption of antimicrobials can be restricted is through more prudent use of antimicrobials.

In the veterinary field as well, there can be great benefits to more targeted use of antimicrobials. The use of antimicrobials in livestock production is very significant at the global level and greatly contributes to the spread of AMR (Rushton et al. 2014). Modern livestock production has become virtually dependent on using antimicrobials since the 1950s. This dependence is due to its use in fighting diseases in the increasingly more intensive animal husbandry as well as growth promoters in the ordinary production. Globally, the growth in the use of antimicrobials is expected to be linked largely to livestock production. As economic growth continues in previously relatively poor countries (e.g., China), the demand for meat grows. It is especially swine and poultry (chicken) production that has grown significantly over the past 20 years. For example,

China has become the world's largest producer of pigs in relatively few years, and the consumption of antimicrobials has increased accordingly. Consequently, Chinese AMR problems have increased in parts of the country. The FAO forecasts that two-thirds of the growth in the consumption of antimicrobials in the coming decades will be linked to livestock production (http://www.fao.org/antimicrobial-resistance/key-sectors/animal-production/en/). Everything thus points to the fact that the use of antimicrobials will not fall in the coming years. On the contrary, antimicrobial consumption will rise despite the various national and international policy initiatives. The AMR problem will remain and may even worsen.

In this book, we have tried to analyze a number of different issues regarding the AMR problem as outlined above. The goal has been to explain why and under what conditions antimicrobials are used in the human and veterinary sectors. In the following sections, we will summarize some of our main conclusions based on the observations highlighted in the various chapters.

12.2 Studying Denmark in a Partially Comparative Perspective

Denmark and Danish experiences have been a continuous theme in this book. One obvious reason for this has been that the research that formed the basis for the analyses has been conducted in Denmark and that the researchers behind the book are all affiliated with the University of Copenhagen and the University of Copenhagen Research Centre for Control of Antibiotic Resistance (UC-care) group. However, the focus on Denmark has also been based on Denmark constituting a special case in relation to the study of AMR. Both in the human and veterinary sectors, consumption of antimicrobials in Denmark is low compared to other countries, as is Denmark's AMR level.

Together with the rest of the Nordic region, Denmark is part of a group of countries characterized by both low consumption of antimicrobials and a low level of AMR cases. This low level applies to both the human area and in connection with livestock production. Considering the need to analyze experiences of how to reduce antimicrobial consumption, the uniquely low level is precisely what makes Denmark suitable as a case.

Some of the studies in this book analyze what the literature refers to as 'prescribing under pressure' (Stivers 2007). Both in the human and veterinary fields, it is well-known that patients or farmers may try to pressure doctors or veterinarians to prescribe antimicrobials, believing that antimicrobials are the only way to improve their own or their animals' health status. Doctors and veterinarians experience how their patients or customers try to persuade them to prescribe more antimicrobials than their immediate professional assessments would warrant.

A number of chapters show that human doctors are acutely aware of the need to limit their prescribing of antimicrobials. Doctors use a range of techniques to convince patients that antimicrobials are unnecessary or to avoid prescribing them. As observed in Chap. 10 (Bank and Rogne), doctors employ humor as one way to convince and communicate to patients that there is no need for prescribing.

Uncertainty about the consequences of not prescribing antimicrobials is an ongoing theme in a number of chapters that focus on doctor–patient relations in the human area. In Chap. 5 (de Oliviera, Flores, and Tembrás), which analyzes doctor–patient relations in Spain, the authors conclude that the Spanish doctors are aware of the Spanish authorities' recommendations that antimicrobials should be prescribed with caution due to the risk of AMR. Nevertheless, a number of doctors stated that in certain situations, they continue to prescribe antimicrobials even though it may not be expressly motivated. The uncertainty about whether the patient's health condition can worsen if no antimicrobials are prescribed can cause doctors to prescribe medicines for purely preventive reasons. The risk of the patient becoming ill (possibly so ill that he or she dies) if the patient does not receive antimicrobials is weighed against the authorities' recommendation to limit consumption (see also Pedersen and Jepsen's discussion in Chap. 9). Similar observations about diagnostic uncertainty can be found in Chap. 10 (Bank and Rogne), which discusses 'liminal zones' when describing the diagnostic state between being ill or not ill.

Diagnoses are rarely unambiguous and doctors must make a concrete assessment about the need for antimicrobials in situations where a precise diagnosis is not possible. Here too, the risk that the patient's condition may worsen affects the doctor's decision to prescribe or not prescribe medication.

As a number of the chapters of the book show, Denmark's agricultural sector, and especially pig producers, has been widely criticized for their use of antimicrobials (Fynbo in Chap. 7; Jensen and Fynbo in Chap. 8). The criticism has been particularly vociferous in the human area because use of antimicrobials in agriculture increases the presence of AMR in the population generally. The possibility of treating patients for diseases is thus reduced as a result of agricultural consumption of antimicrobials.

The reason Denmark presents an interesting case for the study of antimicrobial use in livestock production is that Danish consumption is relatively low in comparison with antimicrobial consumption in other countries. As shown in Chap. 6 (Jensen), Denmark consumes 44 milligrams of antimicrobials per kilogram meat during the process of production. This is comparable to 99 milligrams in France, 204 milligrams in Germany, and 341 milligrams in Italy. In a world where meat production—especially pork—is increasing and where consumption of antimicrobials is growing, these differences in consumption of antimicrobials are very significant.

A number of the chapters of the book analyze various aspects of how antimicrobials are used, especially in pig production. Denmark, especially Danish pig production, comprises an interesting case in an international perspective. This is especially true because Danish pig producers produce mainly for export, making them acutely vulnerable to competitive pressures Yet, Danish farmers can produce pigs in large quantities and at internationally competitive prices without the high consumption of antimicrobials that we find in other countries. As is apparent from Chap. 6 (Jensen), some of the reasons for the comparatively low consumption of antimicrobials among Danish pig farmers lie with a regulatory system that limits the amount of antimicrobials that the individual pig producer must use in production. At the same time, biosecurity is also a concern among Danish pig producers. One of the factors keeping Danish consumption of antimicrobials relatively low is that the pigs are protected against infections, which includes a high level of biosecurity.

12.3 Professions and the One Health Perspective on AMR

Internationally, for the last ten to 15 years, a scientific movement has argued for a 'One Health' perspective in the health field (Kahn 2016). The One Health perspective has also been central to a number of international initiatives to combat AMR, notably in the EU. The One Health perspective implies that both the human and veterinary medical field should be viewed as a single unit. There are several reasons for this.

First, the biological processes that take place in animals and humans are largely parallel and similar. Hence, there can be scientific benefits of linking the two areas that have traditionally been viewed as two separate scientific environments.

Secondly, and particularly relevant to the AMR problem, the importance of zoonoses is growing (Cutler et al. 2010). Zoonoses relate to diseases that can be transmitted between animals and humans. For example, bacteria that might be harmless to animals can be pathogenic to humans. Methicillin-resistant *Staphylococcus aureus*-398 (MRSA)-398 is an example of such zoonosis, where the resistant bacterium from pigs infects humans. MRSA-398 is harmless to the pigs, but problematic for humans.

As a large proportion of global (and Danish) antibiotic consumption occurs in connection with livestock production (especially pigs), the problem of bacteria transfers from animals to humans is highly relevant. Livestock production is a major driver in the development of AMR due to the high consumption of antimicrobials in the sector.

In this book, we have thematized the One Health perspective in different ways. First, we have presented research results that relate to both the human and veterinary fields in Denmark (and in a number of other countries). Regulation of antimicrobial consumption is high in Denmark, both in the human and veterinary fields (see Chap. 6). Livestock producers are subject to different types of regulation to ensure a prudent use of antimicrobials. In the human medicine field, the regulation is primarily aimed at ensuring that doctors and healthcare professionals exert a more prudent approach to prescribing antimicrobials, and there are strict hygiene measures to be applied in areas such as the hospital sector.

Some of the research findings in this book point to the fact that, although there are many professionals in the human and veterinary fields who adhere to the One Health perspective, there remain major differences in the two areas, and in their respective approaches to the use of antimicrobials. Thus, Jensen and Fynbo (Chap. 8), analyzing interviews with experts in the human sciences, veterinarians, and farmers, showed the great differences in perception of pig producers' consumption of antimicrobials. The analysis showed how farmers and their families feel stigmatized as a result of the public debate about the use of antimicrobials, a debate led by experts in human medicine. The observed contradictions between the human and veterinary fields reflect major differences in approaches and perceptions in the two systems.

Some of the chapters in this book link up with the sociological study of professions, and it is from this perspective that some of the doctors' behavior and decision-making related to AMR can be understood and explained. Prescription of antibiotics and combatting AMR takes place in a context embedded in the medical profession's norms for what is good and less good 'doctoring'. Hence, Pedersen, and Jepsen (Chaps. 9 and 11) show how prescription of antimicrobials is embedded in doctors' clinical practices. It is largely the doctors' own experiences and expectations that are important for how they make decisions about prescribing antimicrobials. Pedersen and Jepsen describe the tensions generated between the actual clinical practice and the guidelines that come from the authorities about when and under what conditions to prescribe antimicrobials. Official guidelines are interpreted through doctor's clinical practices.

12.4 Conclusion: The Social Science Perspective

To effectively combat AMR, it is not only essential to comprehend the biological processes whereby bacteria change in interaction with antimicrobial drugs and develop resistance. Excessive use of antibiotics among humans and animals is widely recognized as a crucial factor in causing and exacerbating the problem of resistance, and we need solid knowledge about the factors that lead to overuse. The scientific community should therefore pay equal attention to both the biological and social factors that not only cause resistance but also endanger public health. We need social science to elucidate, for example, how antibiotics are governed and accessed; how officials communicate recommendations and guidelines; which values, beliefs, habits, interpretations, desires, and preferences are exhibited by prescribers and users; how prescribers and users concretely interact, and so on.

One of the motivations behind this volume has been to pay timely attention to such matters by collecting a series of papers written by sociologists, psychologists, and linguists. Our common aim has been to examine the social factors affecting the use of antibiotics among humans and animals. The social scientific methods that have been applied in this pursuit necessarily differ markedly from the kind of clinical and experimental methods commonly employed by natural scientists and medical doctors. Quoting philosopher Alfred Schutz (1953, p. 28): 'It is indeed the particular problem of the social sciences to develop methodological devices for attaining objective and verifiable knowledge of a subjective meaning structure'. The methodological devices used in our studies have included ethnographic observations, qualitative interviews, surveys, document analyses, grammatical analyses, and interactional analyses. Methods such as these have enabled us to scrutinize the subjectivity and human agency that underpin the social factors affecting the use of antibiotics on humans and animals.

More specifically, the use of conversation analysis enabled examinations of the organization of general practitioner consultations with a special focus on patients' situated expressions of concerns and the impact of their concerns on the doctors' subsequent interaction and treatment decision (Chaps. 2 and 4). Several studies used qualitative interviews with doctors to reveal doctors' understandings of what they envisioned as 'good doctoring' in terms of prescription practices (Chap. 9), their regimes for justifying courses of action, which contributes to a relative overuse of antibiotics (Chap. 11), Spanish doctors' accounts of the reasons for an even greater overuse (Chap. 5), and the social stigma experienced by pig farmers and its possible impact on use of antibiotics (Chap. 8). Other studies are anchored in ethnographic observations, or use of such observations in conjunction with semi-structured and possibly also more spontaneous interviews, which have provided insights into pig farmers' concerns and animal surgeons' expert knowledge about antibiotic consumption in the pig industry (Chap. 9), and how general practitioners can handle diagnostic uncertainty and patients' persistent worries during consultations (Chap. 10). Grammatical analysis made it possible to uncover subtle but significant differences in officials' strategic campaign materials advising against excessive use of antibiotics in Denmark, France, and Italy, respectively (Chap. 3). Finally, a combination of document analysis, interviews, and statistical evidence was used to answer the crucial question: How is the use of antibiotics governed in the EU and in Denmark specifically (Chap. 6)?

As can be seen, a range of methodological strategies have been deployed in order to enhance our understanding of the social factors that lead to potential excessive use of antibiotics and what can be done about it. A range of strategies is indeed needed because of the problem's many facets, ranging from legislation and governance, implementation of effective guidelines, economic interests, uneven access, social preferences, and 'glitches' in communication between users and prescribers. This book has by no means covered all the factors related to the excessive use of antibiotics that generates resistance. Such a list would be quite extensive. Rather, our ambition has been to examine some of the most significant factors, such as prescription practices and users' attitudes, and to highlight those factors that indeed require attention and action in order to sustain the benefits of antibiotic treatment in the future.

References

Cutler, S. J., Fooks, A. R., & Van Der Poel, W. H. M. (2010). Public health threat of new, reemerging, and neglected zoonoses in the industrialized world. *Emerging Infectious Diseases, 16*(1), 1–7.

Kahn, L. (2016). *One health and the politics of antimicrobial resistance*. Baltimore, MD: Johns Hopkins University Press.

O'Neill, J. (2014). Antimicrobial resistance: Tackling a crisis for the health and wealth of nations. The Review on Antimicrobial Resistance, Chaired by Jim O'Neill (London, UK).

Rushton, J., Pinto Ferreira, J., & Stärk, K. (2014). Antimicrobial resistance: The use of antimicrobials in the livestock sector. *OECD Food, Agriculture and Fisheries. Papers*, No. 68, OECD Publishing, Paris.

Schutz, A. (1953). Common sense and scientific interpretation of human action. *Philosophy and Phenomenological Research, 14*(1), 1–38.

Stiver, T. (2007). *Prescribing under pressure: Parent-physician conversations and antibiotics*. Oxford: Oxford University Press.

Index[1]

NUMBERS AND SYMBOLS

A

[1] Note: Page numbers followed by 'n' refer to notes.

C. S. Jensen et al. (eds.), *Risking Antimicrobial Resistance*,
https://doi.org/10.1007/978-3-319-90656-0

F

G

H

N

O

P

The manufacturer's authorised representative in the EU is Springer Nature Customer Service Centre GmbH, Europaplatz 3, 69115 Heidelberg, Germany. If you have any concerns regarding our products, please contact ProductSafety@springernature.com

Printed and bound by CPI Group (UK) Ltd, Croydon, CR0 4YY
29/04/2026
02099514-0001